W9-CCS-295

Praise for Previous Editions

"Bakalinsky . . . is the Ferdinand Magellan, the Sir Francis Drake, the Vasco da Gama of San Francisco stairways."

—Paul McHugh, *San Francisco Chronicle*

"A fascinating trek through the sidewalk staircases hidden around the city."

—*The New York Times*

"A wonderfully informative guidebook, custom-made for a city with challenging hills and picture-perfect views . . . chock-full of fascinating details."

—*Travel Books Review*

"Bakalinsky has been scouring the city since the mid-1970s, clambering, walking, exploring tiny alleys and stairways, grand steps, paths and risers that interlace the city."

—*San Diego Union-Tribune*

"Bakalinsky . . . is the reigning queen of walkers in a city that's full of them."

—Joe Yonan, *The Washington Post*

Everything of importance has already been seen
by somebody who didn't notice it.

—*Alfred North Whitehead*

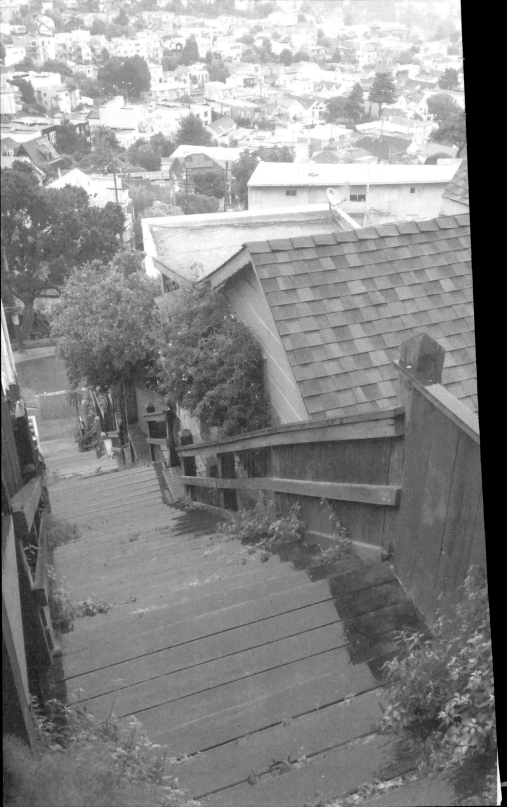

LIVINGSTON PUBLIC LIBRARY
10 Robert H. Harp Drive
Livingston, NJ 07039

Stairway Walks in San Francisco

8th Edition

Mary Burk

with Adah Bakalinsky

 WILDERNESS PRESS ... *on the trail since 1967*

Stairway Walks in San Francisco

3rd edition, 1995
4th edition, 2001
5th edition, 2004
6th edition, 2007
7th edition, 2010
8th edition, 2014

Copyright © 2014 by Mary Burk with Adah Bakalinsky
Editor: Laura Shauger
Maps: Pease Press
Cover and interior photos: Copyright © 2014 by their respective photographers
Cover design: Scott McGrew

Library of Congress Cataloging-in-Publication Data

Bakalinsky, Adah.
  Stairway walks in San Francisco : the joy of urban exploring / Adah Bakalinsky,
Mary Burk.
     pages cm
   ISBN 978-0-89997-749-2 (paperback) — ISBN 0-89997-749-9
   eISBN 978-0-89997-750-8
  1. San Francisco (Calif.)—Tours. 2. Walking—California—San Francisco—Guidebooks. 3. Stairs—California—San Francisco—Guidebooks. I. Burk, Mary. II. Title.
   F869.S33B35 2014
   917.94'6104—dc23
                                2014028303

Manufactured in the United States of America

Published by: **🐾 WILDERNESS PRESS**
            An imprint of Keen Communications, LLC
            PO Box 43673
            Birmingham, AL 35243
            800-443-7227
            info@wildernesspress.com

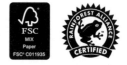

Visit **wildernesspress.com** for a complete listing of our books, and for ordering information.

Distributed by Publishers Group West

Front-cover photos: *Left, top to bottom:* Golden Gate Bridge wave model (Mary Burk);
Onique Stairway, Diamond Heights (Tony Holiday); Sutro Baths Stairway, Lands End
(Tony Holiday). *Right:* Hidden Garden Steps, Golden Gate Heights (Mary Burk).

Frontispiece: Iron Alley Stairway, Twin Peaks Foothills (Mary Burk).

All rights reserved. No part of this book may be reproduced in any form, or by any means
electronic, mechanical, recording, or otherwise, without written permission from the publisher, except for brief quotations used in reviews.

SAFETY NOTICE: Although Wilderness Press and the author have made every attempt to
ensure that the information in this book is accurate at press time, they are not responsible for
any loss, damage, injury, or inconvenience that may occur to anyone while using this book.
The fact that a stairway walk is described in this book does not mean that it will be safe for
you. Note that conditions can change from day to day. Use sound judgment and minimize
your risk on any stairway walk or urban hike by being knowledgeable, prepared, and alert.

Dedication

To Adah Bakalinsky, the Queen of San Francisco Stairways. Adah has entrusted me to continue her book, and I am humbled and honored to do so. We have enjoyed taking all of the walks and further ramblings in this edition together, and I hope you will enjoy taking these walks as much as we did.

And to new walkers and those trying out something like this for the first time. I am so happy knowing you are about to take on a small, simple adventure, and I wish you a most fortuitous, serendipitous amble.

San Francisco is enlivened by its great architecture, spirited by its vibrant and individual citizens, and as always, it quietly whispers its history and natural beauty to those walking about and listening. It is this magic through movement that brought Adah's walks together. The walks have a rhythm all their own, and like a dance, or a pattern, each were formed by what feels right in stride. We're happy to have you along!

However, Adah and I both know that as soon as something is captured or noticed, it changes. And places change too, night or day, and through various weather—and so everyone experiences different thoughts, ideas, and feelings along their own paths. So as you get out there, know that you are in good company; walking is the type of activity most folks can enjoy, and you all are just who this book was tailor-made for. Best wishes to you as you continue exploring, everywhere you go.

Thank you, dear readers. Now watch your step, and mind the path.

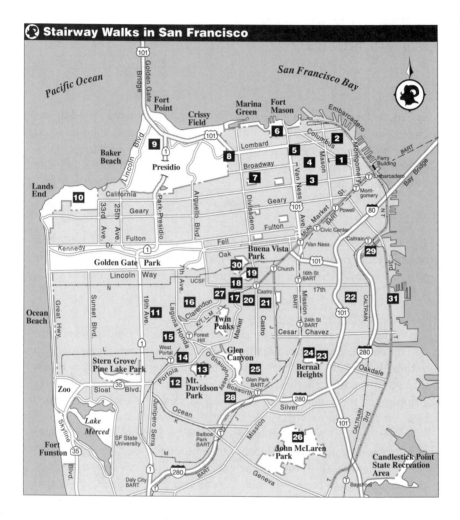

Stairway Walks in San Francisco

Contents

Acknowledgments

So much of this book came into being because of the work, sweat, tenacity, and beauty of its original author and the amazing, wonderful people who have helped, encouraged, and laughed with Adah along her way. Thanks to Charles Brock for the stairways index (see the appendix) and to Ben Pease for his work on maps for the seventh and eighth editions.

Adah's network of connections and contacts is still very active, and the Hidden Garden Steps group took its community improvement projects to Facebook to promote them to a broader audience. Thanks to artists Aileen Barr and Colette Crutcher for beautifying another Golden Gate Heights stairway; the neighborhood grows more magical with each mosaic. The Glen Canyon, Corona Heights, and Dogpatch neighborhoods, among others, have also proved to be valuable resources for news in the area.

So many people enjoy this city and express themselves online that inspiration was always at hand digitally to keep me inspired even when I had to be indoors. Thanks for inspiration specifically from Tony Holiday, Jake Sigg, and Julian Michelucci, whose dedication to stairways and hiking around San Francisco reaches many others with similar interests. Thanks are also due to Mister SF, for his local San Francisco blog and points of interest, and to Dave Schweisguth, whose hill updates for the mainland and the surrounding islands helped me take a new look at the growing list of hills in the city, named and unnamed.

When I take each walk again and as the seasons change, I continue to find beautiful, sustaining vistas at lookouts and on hilltops and try to keep my eyes peeled for partly hidden gems to look out for around any bend. And after hopping around town every weekend the past year, visiting all of the stairways, rewalking the walks, taking notes and snapping photos, I love the city and its transportation agencies even more. Thank you, SF MUNI (Municipal Transportation Agency), for having GPS triangulation and reliable schedule times, and thank you, San Francisco Police Department and Department of Parking and Traffic, for not towing my car this year; I'm still paying off the parking tickets.

I am so deeply humbled and honored to help continue this exploration of the city with Adah. Thanks to the San Francisco Department of Public Works for their installation of the plaque at the Adah Bakalinsky Stairway,

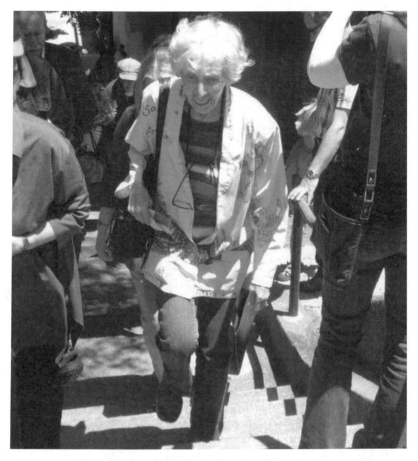

Adah ascends the stairway named in her honor at its 2012 dedication.   *Mike Jones*

although it was recently stolen. Hopefully the replacement won't be as tempting, and we look forward to its arrival and installation.

Thanks mainly though to Adah Bakalinsky, who is my friend. There are so many words, but fitting them together doesn't compare to the silent music that makes up the rhythm of a walk. Adah often mentions that there is music—like jazz—in a walk and that it's always open to interpretation. So for our next walk, since it will be time spent in the company of a friend, I suspect we might try a little stride piano, followed by a shuffle, and then a little walking down the keys, but we will have to play it all by ear.

Thanks also for personal time with Weggie and June Bug and to Jason for never letting me forget my deadlines. Thanks also to my mother and her parents, who raised me to appreciate beauty in life, in others, and in myself.

Foreword

As a former mayor of San Francisco and now as lieutenant governor of California, my work includes civic management, promoting civic pride, and honoring civic-minded individuals. Ten years ago, as mayor, I honored Adah Bakalinsky for her work in bringing neighborhoods together through her book, *Stairway Walks in San Francisco*. Now, San Francisco City Guides organizes stairway walks every year in May to get people out to enjoy all that this wonderful city has to offer.

I recognize the benefits individuals gain through walking, and I also understand the benefits a city neighborhood gains when residents work together to improve their surroundings. San Francisco is seeing a resurgence in civic pride around its stairways, as neighbors and volunteers come together to maintain them. Artists are also now turning stairways into canvases (such as the magical Moraga Stairway and the similarly stunning Hidden Garden Steps), beautifying the city even further.

Stairways in San Francisco neighborhoods bring people together by giving residents a public connection to their surroundings. It's a state of mind that connects citizens to the public agencies that maintain our public parks and open areas, like the Department of Public Works (DPW) and the Golden Gate National Recreation Area. It also allows individuals to become more engaged and brings brand new groups together. It enables pride to be built in our communities throughout the city.

Growing up in San Francisco, I enjoyed walking in and among the hills of the city. Thankfully, there were stairways to provide a shortcut when I trekked up and down these steep slopes. Since walking is really the best way to get to know and experience San Francisco, these stairs provide a helpful and often breathtaking view of our city.

In 2012 the San Francisco DPW dedicated a stairway in the Upper Haight neighborhood to Adah. That stairway bears her name to honor her work and the influence she had in showing San Franciscans how important these stairways are to all of us. I am also proud and honored to write this foreword for this eighth edition for which Mary Burk has taken the reins.

Stairway Walks in San Francisco retains the city's history, appreciates the city's beauty, and most importantly, encourages healthy activity. Adah's walks introduced me to three secrets, and I encourage you to discover them on a San Francisco stairway walk of your own:

- *Serendipity:* You never know whom you may meet.
- *Well-being:* Walking up and down stairs is good for the heart and mind.
- *Stupendous views:* The secret vistas at the top of many of San Francisco's stairways are simply breathtaking.

—Gavin Newsom
Lieutenant Governor of California
July 2014

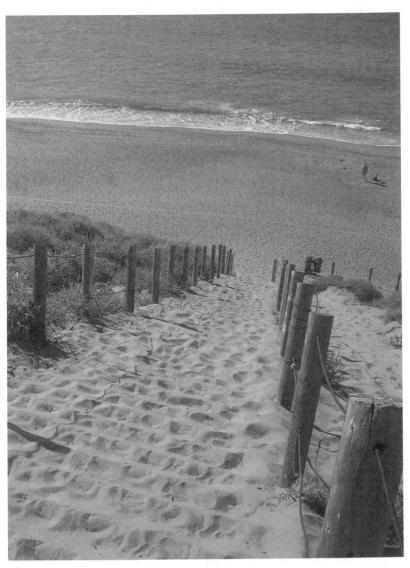

Sand ladder at Baker Beach *Tony Holiday*

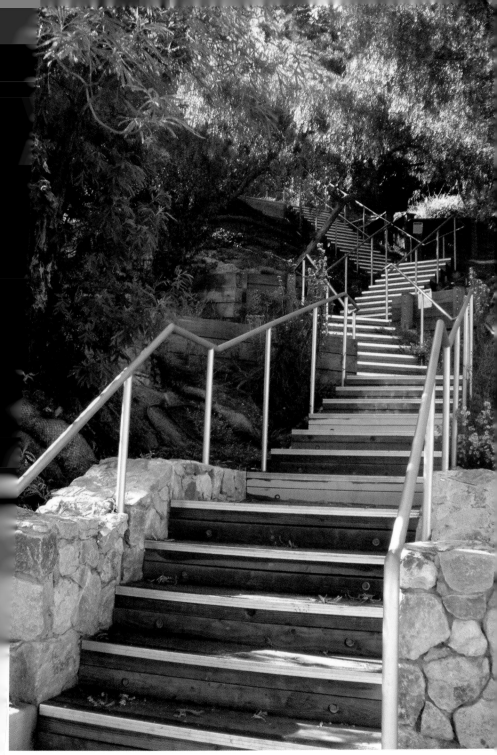

Buena Vista Park, Upper Haight (Walk 30)

Marion Gregoire

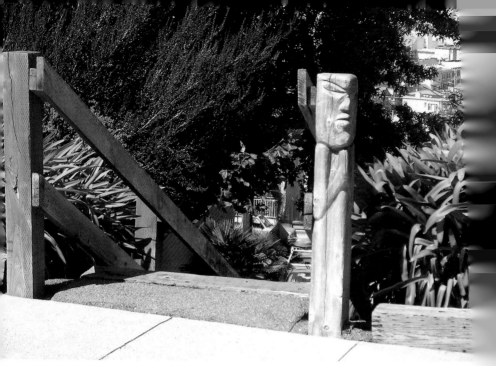

Franconia Stairway, Bernal Heights East (Walk 23)   *Tony Holiday*

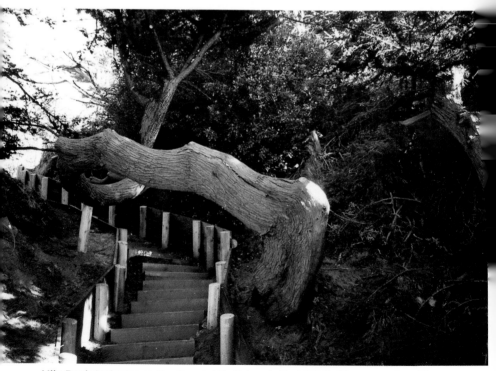

Mile Rock Stairway on the Coastal Trail, Lands End (Walk 10)   *Peter Nagy*

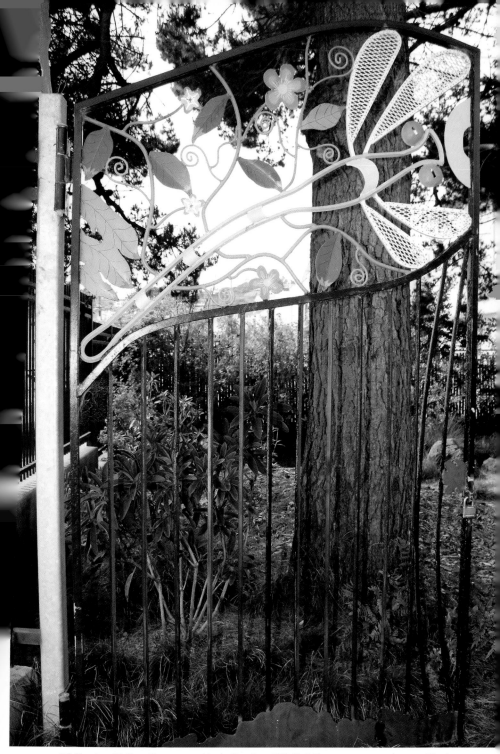

Visitacion Valley Greenway Herb Garden (Walk 26)

Annette Hovie

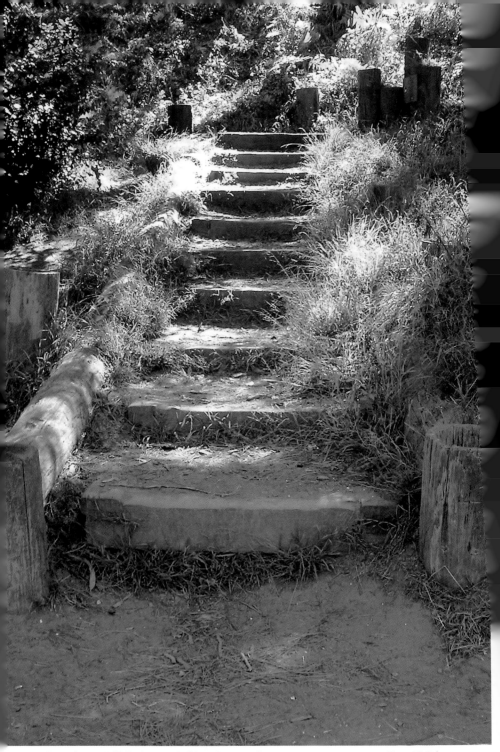

Strawberry Hill Stairway, Golden Gate Park

Tony Holiday

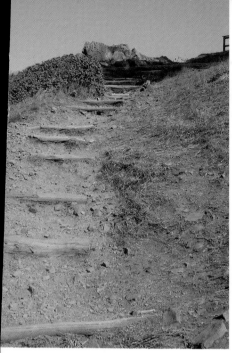

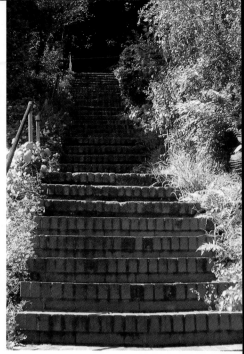

Tank Hill Stairway, Twin Peaks
Foothills (Walk 17)   *Tony Holiday*

Jack Early Park Stairway, Telegraph Hill
(Walk 2)   *Tony Holiday*

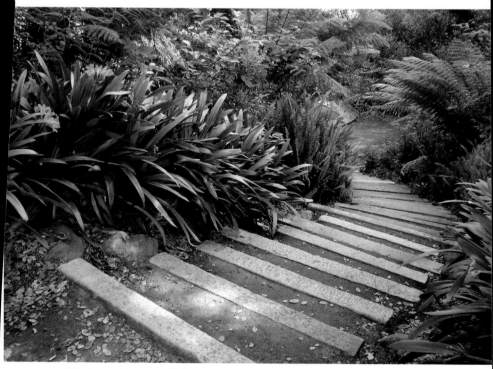

AIDS Memorial Grove Stairway, Golden Gate Park   *Tony Holiday*

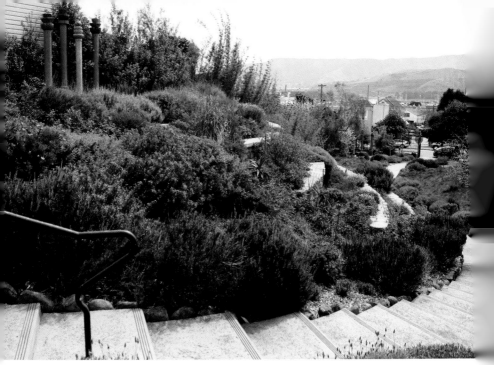

Visitacion Valley Greenway (Walk 26)   *Annette Hovie*

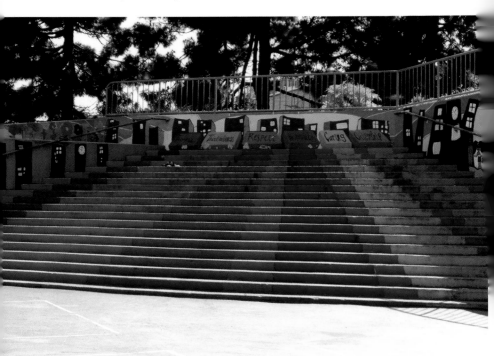

McKinley School Playground, Corona Heights (Walk 19)   *Adah Bakalinsky*

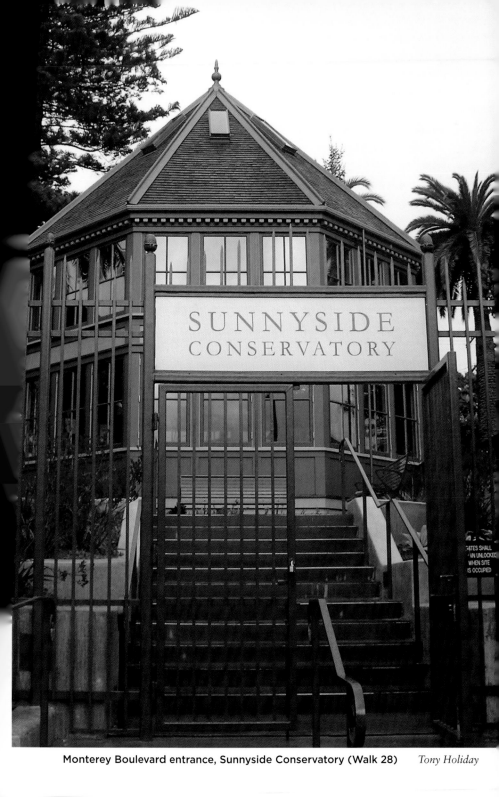

Monterey Boulevard entrance, Sunnyside Conservatory (Walk 28)   *Tony Holiday*

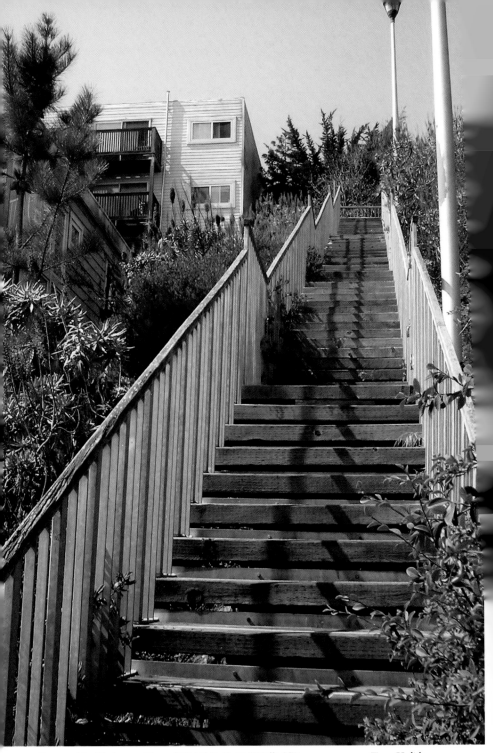

Esmeralda Stairway, Bernal Heights East (Walk 23)   *Tony Holiday*

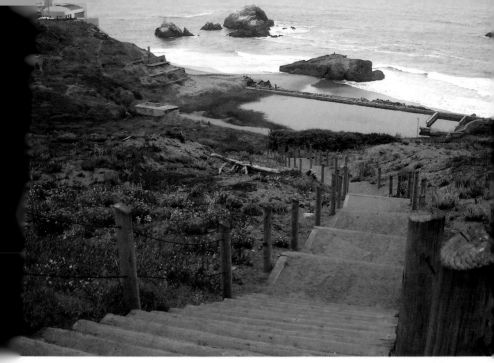

Sutro Baths Stairway, Lands End (Walk 10) *Tony Holiday*

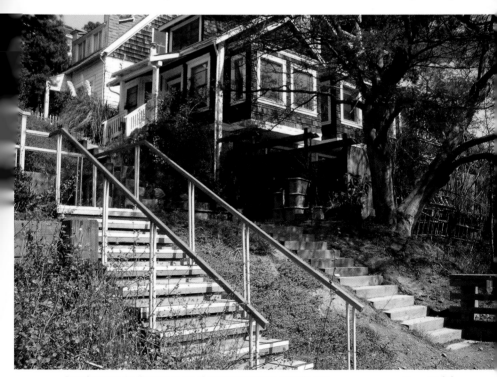

Powhattan Stairway, Bernal Heights West (Walk 24) *Tony Holiday*

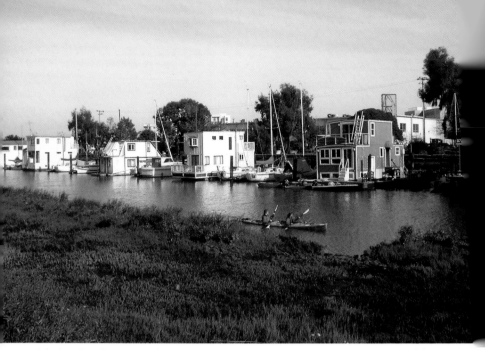

Mission Creek Marina, The Blue Greenway (Walk 29)   *Tony Holiday*

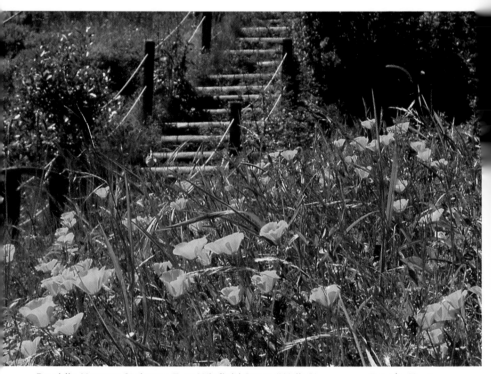

Presidio Nursery Stairway, Fort Winfield Scott (Walk 9)   *Presidio Trust*

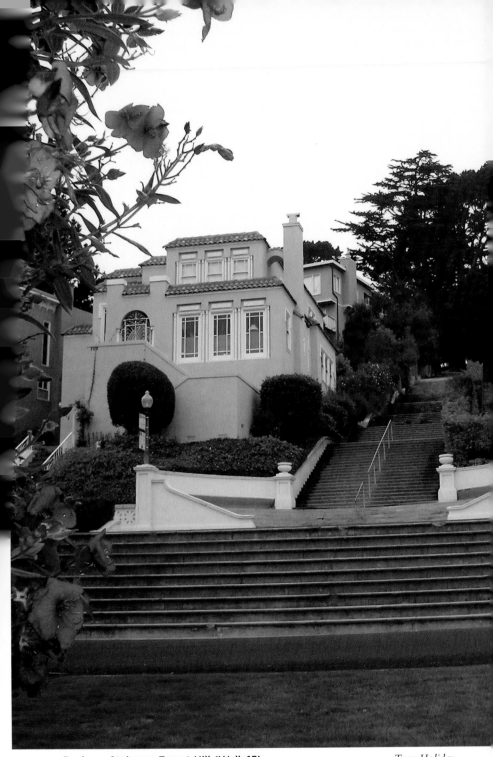

Pacheco Stairway, Forest Hill (Walk 15)

Tony Holiday

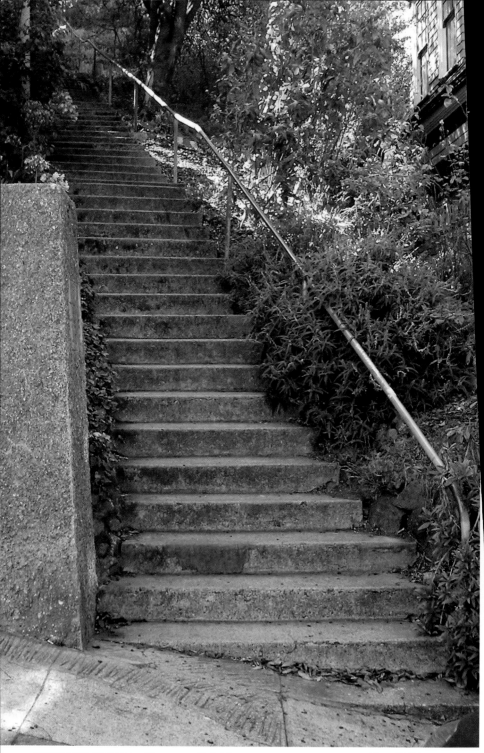

Farnsworth Stairway, Parnassus Heights   *Tony Holiday*

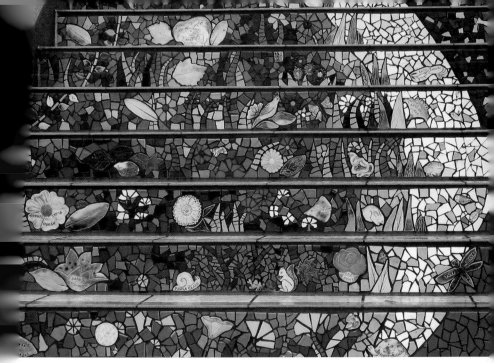

Mosaic tile stairway at 16th Ave. and Moraga (Walk 11)   *James Charney*

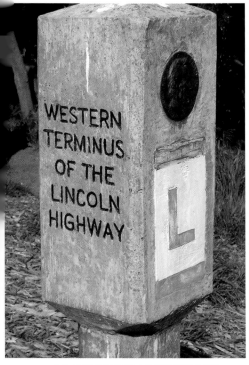

WESTERN TERMINUS OF THE LINCOLN HIGHWAY

L

Lincoln Highway memorial post
(Walk 10)   *Tony Holiday*

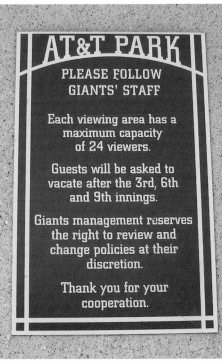

AT&T PARK

PLEASE FOLLOW
GIANTS' STAFF

Each viewing area has a
maximum capacity
of 24 viewers.

Guests will be asked to
vacate after the 3rd, 6th
and 9th innings.

Giants management reserves
the right to review and
change policies at their
discretion.

Thank you for your
cooperation.

Free View sign at AT&T Park (Walk 29)
Tony Holiday

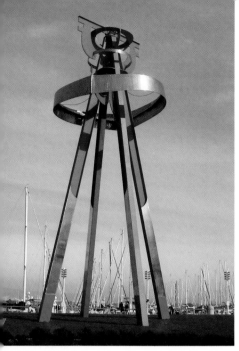

Mark di Suvero's *Sea Change*
(Walk 29)   *Tony Holiday*

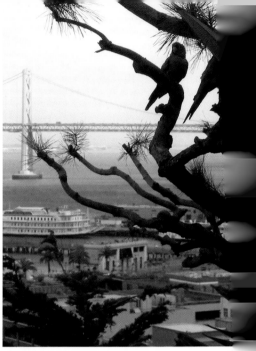

A view of the Bay from Calhoun Terrace
(Walk 1)   *James Charney*

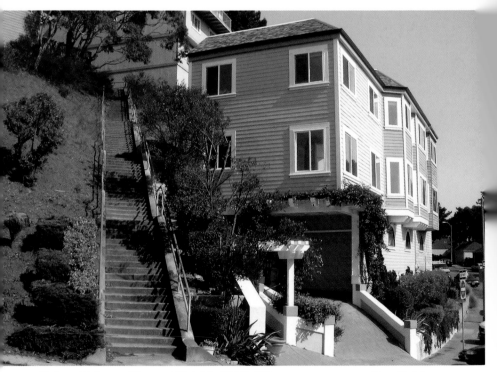

Onique Stairway, Diamond Heights (Walk 25)   *Tony Holiday*

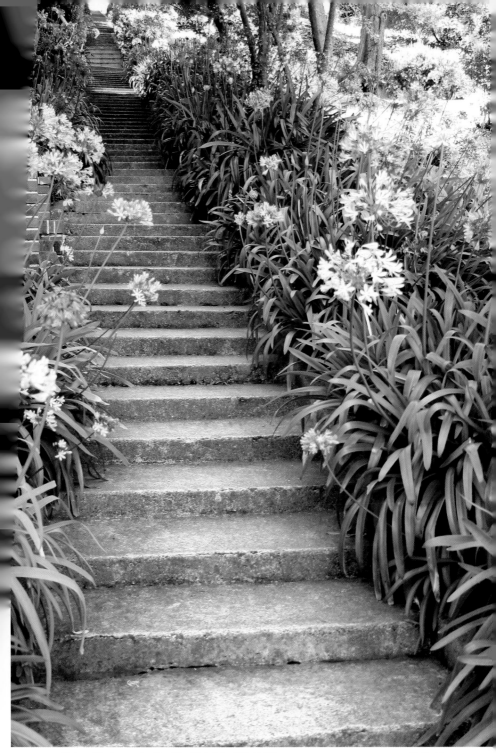

Baker Stairway in Pacific Heights (Walk 7)

Polly Gates

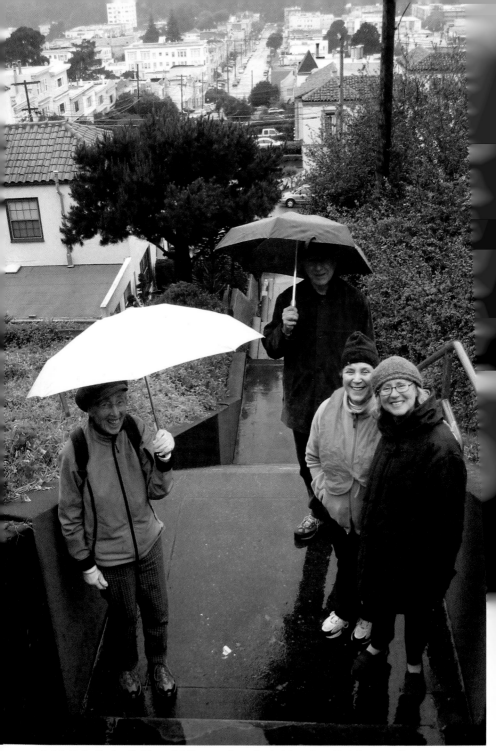

Adah Bakalinsky (left) and fellow walkers in Golden Gate Heights (Walk 11)
James Charney

Introduction

I've taken the direct path and arrived at a glorious dinner party. Around me are notable walkers from across the globe, hailing from past and present. They are gathered here to discuss the topic of urban exploring, in a city that is undoubtedly quite walkable, where they will meet and greet the most elite fleet of feet on a landing halfway up a staircase in San Francisco.

Our host is Adah Bakalinsky, the queen of the city's stairways. Our crowned sovereign reigns because her walks knit together via vertical path, and her strolls, known far and wide, quickly spark some of the best conversations among those gathered. Time passes splendidly, with lively conversations percolating among all the perambulatory party patrons. A discourse of wrong turns, happy happenstances, and nature's beauty is exchanged and enjoyed anew, electrifying the air. Suddenly, the shuffling of anxious, happy feet becomes noticeable when someone suggests a stairway walk, and enthusiasm quickly enlivens the group to rise to their feet and begin. As I wake up, I realize I have been kicking the covers in excitement—as I too am literally ready to jump out of bed. So I do.

I had the pleasure of meeting Adah 15 years ago at the San Francisco Public Main Library. I am so glad I told Adah how much I enjoyed her walks back then, and I am so glad too that we've had so many good walks together as well. Like Adah, I am blessed to live here, and we both are humbled by the friendly strangers and locals we meet daily, especially when we let a walk take us on a new adventure around town or up a familiar stairway and hill in any sort of weather.

Adah sees how stairways knit our neighborhoods together, embracing our various little enclaves strung along over hill and yonder dale. My own interest in the city took on a new dimension once I started exploring it through Adah's stairway walks, and I never doubt what treasures I can still discover when escalating by foot, tread, and riser to the next platform up ahead. I am honored to continue this work for Adah, happily highlighting all the little gems this city wants to share with us. Also, ascending ambulation is absolutely awesome, but let me walk that back—what I mean is, I enjoy walking up (and down) stairs too, so it's a great pleasure to continue Adah's stairway walks in this newest, eighth edition.

I have added two new walks and updated all 29 existing walks with new information, where changes or improvements that impacted the walk or its landmarks occurred since the last edition. Look for the Adah Bakalinsky Stairway in Walk 30 (The Good View). Imagine what once was a brawling bowery and bustling immigrant community now scraped away from tiny Irish Hill in Walk 31 (The Serendipity Slipknot), which still includes one stairway.

But before we get started, and for those of you who have not been on this journey with Adah before, let me first say a bit more about where you are at least reading about walking, if you are not already moving, around there, or here—right now.

All civilizations have built stairs, and the oldest still preserved date back to 7000 BCE. The Greeks and, before them, the Egyptians, and then, before them, Phoenicians, Sumerians, and Elamites too, used steps and terraces to farm, travel, pray, and even practice sacrifice. Moving up was desired and beneficial, unless you were, of course, an unwilling sacrifice.

Because stairs have been used for so long, their inventor is probably lost to the ages. However, ever since those first unknown walkers pressed their soles into soft earth and yielding roots in the hill ahead, and until they clambered onward and upward just to get where they wanted to go or to escape what they wanted to get away from, stairs were just waiting to be discovered.

Classical stairway design influenced European design, from Italy with Palladio to France with Nicolas Blondel, the standard design for tread and riser became part of architectural treatises and materials widely adopted and used from the 17th through the 20th centuries in both America and Europe, and these designs still influence public and private stairway design in cities worldwide.

San Francisco is a "walking city." Built upon 43 hills, with another 28 thrown in for good measure, the city is surrounded by the Bay on the east, the Pacific Ocean to the west, a peninsula to the south, and the Golden Gate to the north. Within these confines, however, variety is constant. Light and water combine to produce striking effects on bridges and buildings throughout the day; and at sunset, beams of light dramatize the hills and sides of houses, casting colors like Cézanne. Mirrored tiles and windows glitter like mosaic tiles on the magic stairway at Moraga and 16th Avenue, and its fantastic new sibling at 16th and Kirkham, the Hidden Garden Steps. Come out at sunrise, sunset, in the fog, or in the sun, and take a walk.

Hills and mountains were made to be climbed, and stairways make it easier to traverse them. The hills accelerate changes in perspective as you walk around corners or circle the ridges. Landmarks recede and

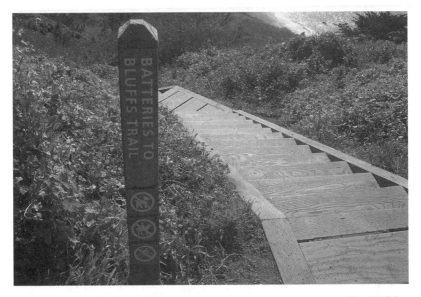

Batteries to Bluff Stairway (Walk 9)   *Tony Holiday*

suddenly emerge in a landscape abounding in inclines and angled streets. The Mt. Sutro TV Tower viewed from the mid-Sunset District is a beautiful sky sculpture; from the Sutro Urban Forest, it looks like a ship in space. From Ashbury Heights, it looks pedestrian. Then it appears large again, and within touching distance from the Outer Sunset District; now walk two blocks toward it, and it appears distant and small.

The streets of San Francisco range from comparatively flat, such as Irving, to almost vertical, such as sections of Duboce, Filbert, and Duncan. The city's founders and developers found grading the streets on hills a primary obstacle when converting San Francisco from a tent town into a city of timbered houses. Some of the hills were completely demolished in the process; others were cut into without much planning. When the task seemed insurmountable, the "street" ended. Our streets were pummeled and pushed into rectangular grids familiar from the East Coast, but inappropriate for our terrain. Paved streets often follow the contours of hills, but the stairways allow a direct vertical approach from one street to another. They provide accessibility to public transportation; they provide safety in case of fire; and they limit degradation of the land. Plus everyone loves a shortcut.

Within the city limits, there are more than 671 stairways of all descriptions: crooked, straight, short, long, concrete, wood, balustraded, unadorned, narrow, and wide. Some of the stairways are not as easily identified; look on the sidewalk to see if the stairway name is given there—sometimes it is even if a stairway does not have a sign. Sometimes their names are assumed, much like those of some lesser-known hills in the city are.

These walks are designed for the curious walker who loves to explore. Each walk takes between two and two and a half hours if you enjoy all the sights, scents, and sounds along the way. Walks in more well-known neighborhoods like Pacific Heights and Telegraph Hill are here, as are walks in less well-known neighborhoods like Eureka Valley, Edgehill, and Dogpatch. All of the walks offer visual interest in the immediate setting and surrounding areas and also often produce new organic stories shared by neighbors near the stairs.

The walks are best enjoyed at a pace considered reasonable or steady— give yourself time to look around. The pace of a walk is almost as important as its length or difficulty since everyone needs to give themselves more time to think and imagine. Here, your destination is the walk, so you've already arrived. By slowing down, walking half as fast, and taking in what surrounds you, time is the bonus, the joy is in the moving, and the reward is in the path.

The beginning point of each walk can be reached by public transportation (call 311 or visit **sfmuni.com** for routes and schedules) or the free PresidiGo shuttle for the Presidio (call 415-561-5300 or visit **presidio.gov /tenants/transit/downtown.htm**). Buses are available at several points of most walks, and alternate routes are occasionally suggested for specific reasons. Some of the walks are quite strenuous, but the rewards of stupendous views and delightful discoveries justify the effort.

In order to appreciate the scaffolding of the city and the variety of neighborhoods within a whistle's call, I've included some graceful links to other walks in other neighborhoods that can be traversed comfortably in a single session. Look for these recommendations in each walk's Further Rambling section.

Using the map given for a particular walk is helpful if you can locate yourself; use the map legend, and orient yourself on the map and the points of the compass. Each walk's quick-step instructions correspond to the numbered circles on its map. Orienting yourself will help you know which direction you are facing when you can't see the sun rising in the east or setting in the west, when it is foggy, for instance. Look for street numbers and landmarks too, and always watch for traffic. Always look carefully when crossing streets, and remember drivers may not see you if they are distracted, so do be careful.

I suggest that walkers carry the following gear to make their adventure more comfortable: binoculars, a city map, a compass, water, fruit, sunscreen, and layered clothing, especially long pants and long-sleeved shirts for walks where vegetation may hide poison oak. I use the directions left and right, but also the compass points (north, east, south, and west) to provide additional assurance. I also highly recommend the map "Nature in the City," which is available for free from the Department of Recreation and Parks. It shows the parks and other green areas in the city.

This edition includes an updated list of every public stairway in San Francisco (see the appendix). Charles Brock has walked every public stairway and every step in San Francisco, and his efforts doubled the previous list. We added one new stairway to this edition's list and are on the lookout for new public stairways to add as necessary. The descriptions in the walks were up-to-date at publication time. However, neighborhoods continually evolve. If you find discrepancies, please inform Wilderness Press.

Map Legend

IIIIIIIIIIIIIIIIII	Featured stairway	❶	Start/end of walk
▬▬▬	Featured street	❷	Intermediate points
▬ ▬ ▬ ▬	Featured path	🅰	Picnic area
············	Alternate route	▬	Building
IIIIIIIIIIIIIIIIII	Other stairway	•	Point of interest
─ ─ ─ ─	Other path	⊶	Gate
────────	Street	▲	Hill
N ⊕	Rail transit route and station	200	Address
▢	Park or preserve	⬆	North indicator
▨	Other open space		
▭	Body of water		

Treasures & Digressions

Yerba Buena Cove, Telegraph Hill & Chinatown

Early-18th-century Spanish explorers designated three important foci in the city: religious,
Mission Dolores; military, the Presidio; and commercial, Yerba Buena Cove. On this walk, we'll explore the
commercial area.

You will see buildings that were erected on the edge of
the shoreline along the middle third of Yerba Buena Cove, now
the financial and commercial section of San Francisco. You walk
toward Portsmouth Square, which was the center of the Pueblo of
Yerba Buena and now is the center of Chinatown; you continue to the
slopes of Telegraph Hill where the 19th-century waterfront workers lived.
You may feel you are traveling through a land of plaques in this walk
and Walk 2. The northeast part of the city is a small, concentrated area
where the early Spanish commercial history of San Francisco began. The
well-written plaques don't overburden you with a multitude of facts; they
include just enough to stir up your imagination.

The Gold Rush to California was the Outward Bound of the
1800s, the 19th-century rite of passage. It took all of a person's ingenu-
ity, statesmanship, business acumen, and physical stamina to survive. San
Francisco, the entry point for people coming overland by wagon and
around Cape Horn by ship, had a population of approximately 450 at
the first census count in 1847 and approximately 20,000 by the end of
1849. Gradually, as more families arrived in the city, social services were
organized; schools, libraries, and churches were opened; lectures, operas,
concerts, readings, and theater were offered.

Telegraph Hill, at 284 feet in elevation, used to extend east to Battery, near the edge of the Bay, making it difficult to unload cargo. After
the east slope of the hill was quarried, it extended just to the west side of
Sansome. Dock workers living in the small cottages along the hillside used
a stairway to go to and from work. During the late 19th and early 20th
centuries, artists, writers, and actors lived on the hill. Junius Booth of the

(Continued on page 10)

7

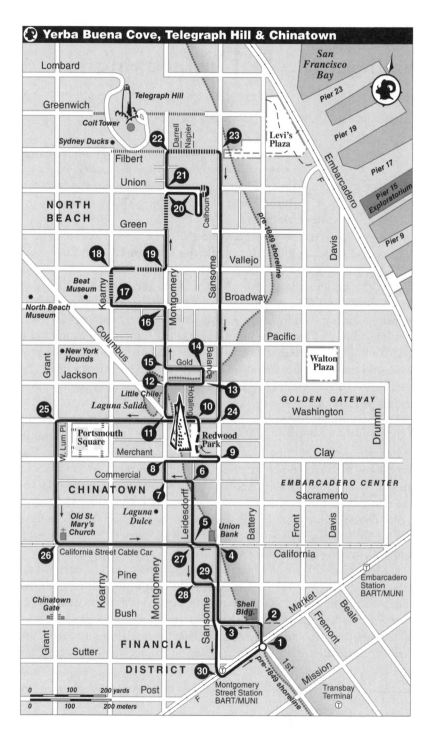

Yerba Buena Cove, Telegraph Hill & Chinatown

Lombard

Greenwich

Telegraph Hill

Coit Tower

Sydney Ducks

Filbert

Union

NORTH
BEACH

Green

Beat
Museum

North Beach
Museum

Columbus

New York
Hounds

Jackson

Little Chile
Laguna Salida

Portsmouth
Square

Merchant

Commercial

CHINATOWN

Old St.
Mary's
Church

Laguna
Dulce

California Street Cable Car

Pine

Bush

Chinatown
Gate

FINANCIAL

Sutter

DISTRICT

Post

Grant

Kearny

Montgomery

Sansome

Darrell
Napier
Calhoun

Vallejo

Broadway

Pacific

Gold

Hotaling

Balance

Washington

Clay

Redwood
Park

Sacramento

Union
Bank

California

Battery

Front

Davis

Leidesdorff

Shell
Bldg.

Market

San
Francisco
Bay

Pier 23

Pier 19

Levi's
Plaza

Pier 17

Pier 15
Exploratorium

Embarcadero

Pier 9

pre-1849 shoreline

Davis

Walton
Plaza

GOLDEN GATEWAY

Drumm

EMBARCADERO CENTER

Embarcadero
Station
BART/MUNI

Beale

Fremont

Montgomery
Street Station
BART/MUNI

1st

Mission

pre-1849 shoreline

Transbay
Terminal

0   100   200 yards
0   100   200 meters

QUICK-STEP INSTRUCTIONS

1. Begin at 1st and Market. Cross Market to the intersection of Battery and Bush.

2. Left on Bush.

3. Right on Sansome to California. Cross to far side.

4. Left on California to Leidesdorff.

5. Right on Leidesdorff to Commercial.

6. Left on Commercial to Montgomery.

7. Right on Montgomery to Clay.

8. Right on Clay, a few yards past Redwood Park to Two Transamerica Center to see the Niantic plaque.

9. Return to walk through the park to Sansome. (The Washington St. gate is open Monday–Friday, during business hours. During this time, you can exit directly to Washington.)

10. Left on Washington to Montgomery.

11. Right on Montgomery to Jackson.

12. Right on Jackson to Balance.

13. Left on Balance to Gold.

14. Left on Gold to Montgomery.

15. Right (north) on Montgomery to Broadway.

16. Left on Broadway to Kearny.

17. Right to ascend Kearny Stairway to Vallejo.

18. Right to descend Vallejo Stairway to Montgomery.

19. Left to ascend Montgomery Stairway to Union.

20. Right turn into Union cul-de-sac. Descend stairway on left to walkway. Ascend stairway on right to Calhoun Terrace and turn left.

21. Return to Montgomery and turn right to Filbert.

22. Right on Filbert to descend stairway to Sansome.

23. Right on Sansome to Washington.

24. Right on Washington to right side of Grant to see No. 823 (some merchandise belonging to the adjoining boutique may hide the number, but it's there).

25. Left (south) on Grant to California.

26. Left on California to Leidesdorff.

27. Right on Leidesdorff to Pine.

28. Left on Pine to Sansome.

29. Right on Sansome to Market.

30. Left on Market to 1st and your beginning.

(Continued from page 7)

famous theater family lived at No. 5 Calhoun Terrace. Writer Charles Warren Stoddard spent part of his childhood here at No. 287 Union. The hill became a special province due in part to its isolated site.

WALK FACTS

Telegraph Hill was known as "Loma Alta" under Spanish rule. Its current name comes from the installation in 1850 of a semaphore flag system, which allowed ship crews to telegraph about the goods they had on board to those waiting for the cargo.

In 1846, 200 people lived around one tiny adobe on the shoreline that was proclaimed Portsmouth Square, named for the ship that Captain John Montgomery brought into the cove that year. Yerba Buena Cove was renamed San Francisco that same year after the Mexican-American War, and its shoreline street, Montgomery, was named for the captain.

Founded in the 1840s, Chinatown in San Francisco is the largest of its kind outside of China and the oldest Chinatown in North America. It was rebuilt around Portsmouth Square in 1910 in the stylized architecture the area is known for today.

Come to Chinatown and stay for the Lunar New Year, which falls between January and March. Enjoy an early morning stroll through the markets and shops to take in the invigorating hustle and bustle.

Bus Routes & Parking

PUBLIC TRANSPORTATION: The many streetcars, buses, or Metro lines that run along Market Street are useful for reaching this route. For MUNI bus information, call 311 (outside San Francisco, call 415-701-2311).

PARKING: There is metered street parking available; metered parking is usually available for up to an hour, and free street parking is usually allowed for up to two hours. But also look for street-cleaning times posted in the neighborhood to avoid getting ticketed or towed.

WALK 1 DESCRIPTION

⬗ Begin at Market and 1st St. (the first street west of Yerba Buena Cove, now about a half mile from the Ferry Building and the Bay). An interpretive plaque is embedded in the sidewalk. No. 525 Market, the Cushman-Wakefield Building, straddles the shoreline. During the week, visitors can see the current art exhibits in the lobby.

⬗ Cross Market to its intersection with Battery and Bush. At the corner near the *Mechanics Monument,* another embedded plaque shows a map of Yerba Buena Cove. The monument was commissioned in 1894 by Peter Donahue to honor his father, James Donahue, founder of Union Iron Works. The foundry, one of the most successful firms in early San Francisco, was located on Harrison, which provided easy access to the Bay. Douglas Tilden, known as the Michelangelo of the West, sculpted the figures on the monument. Although he had been deaf since childhood, his talent was recognized early, and he was able to study in Paris.

⬗ Cross Battery at Bush to see another building that straddles the cove—the 29-story Shell Building at No. 100 Bush. George Pelham designed and built it in 1929–1930. Consistent restoration work has preserved its Art Deco detailing. The shell motif is repeated in the transom, as a light fixture, and in the lobby. At night, the building is suffused with a golden light. Walk over to No. 130 Bush to see the Heineman Building, an anomaly and a curiosity. It is the narrowest building in San Francisco; three steps into the lobby, and you are almost in the elevator.

⬗ Continue west to Sansome, and then north to California. The Union Bank straddles the shoreline at No. 400 California. It was originally the Bank of California, founded in 1864 by William Ralston and O. J. Mills. Bliss and Faville, famous for their classical government buildings, designed it in 1907–08 in Beaux Arts style, beautiful and elegant, but everything is oversized, perfect for a display of power and wealth, and it makes you feel like a Lilliputian. (Two of their other buildings of note and that Adah is very fond of are the Convent of the Sacred Heart School [1912] and the St. Francis Hotel [1904, rebuilt in 1907].) The 21-story tower incorporated into the bank structure was designed by Anshen and Allen in 1967. The integration of the old and new edifices is considered one of the most successful and aesthetic in the city, and the coffered ceiling is elegant. Two plaques near the entrance of the bank provide a fine introduction to a visit of the interior to which you are welcome. The historic exhibit downstairs has artifacts from the early days of gold mining, including a cabinet with pieces of gold that were exchanged for money. The museum is open Monday through Friday.

▪ Continue west (to your left) on California to the intersection of Leidesdorff, which marks the old shoreline. It is named for Captain William Alexander Leidesdorff, a prosperous businessman, linguist, and master of the ship *Julia Ann,* which carried Hawaiian sugar that was traded for California hides. Leidesdorff also was active in fur trading with the Russians at Fort Ross. He settled in Yerba Buena in 1838 and built the City Hotel at Kearny and Clay and a warehouse on the beach at California and Leidesdorff. The captain, born of Danish and African ancestry in the Virgin Islands, died of cholera in 1848 at the age of 36.

▪ Walk to your right through Leidesdorff toward Sacramento. Read the plaque that details the history of What Cheer House (left side of the street), a hotel built by R. B. Woodward in 1852. He later added a private library and museum for guests, an unusual facility for hotels to offer. Captain Ulysses S. Grant stayed there in 1854. (Woodward's Gardens near Mission and 14th St. was the popular outdoor resort in the city in the 1860s.) Laguna Dulce, a freshwater pond fed by a Nob Hill stream, was situated a half block away at Montgomery and Sacramento. It was also the site of a Native American sweat lodge.

▪ Continue on Leidesdorff to Commercial St. (You are now standing in water.) Turn left and walk to Montgomery to stand in the place where Captain John B. Montgomery sailed up in the USS *Portsmouth,* in 1846, to claim the Pueblo of Yerba Buena (established in 1839) for the United States. The Mexican government acceded. It was a quiet takeover. The Pacific Heritage Museum at No. 608 Commercial (free and open Thursday–Saturday, 10 a.m.–4 p.m.) has exhibits relating to Chinese history and customs.

▪ Continue on Montgomery to Clay. Read the plaque on the side of No. 550, at the southeast corner where the Bank of Italy was located in 1904. In the early years, the bank used solicitors to sell accounts. Across the street is the Transamerica Pyramid. The original building on this site was the 1853 Montgomery Block, affectionately known as the Monkey Block. Designed and built by architect Gordon Cummings for Henry Halleck, it was also known as Halleck's Folly because it cost $2 million. Four stories high, it had a fish market, grocery, and the Saloon Bank Exchange Bar, where bankers transacted business. In later years, law offices and the largest law library in the area were located in the Monkey Block. Sun Yat-sen, founder of the Chinese Nationalist movement, had his office here during his exile, around 1911. In the 1920s and 1930s, artists, writers, and dancers rented studio and living quarters here. Among them were Pietro Mezzara, the sculptor who made the first statue of Abraham Lincoln; George Sterling, the poet; and Ann Munstock, who brought modern dance to San Francisco from Germany.

◢ The Monkey Block withstood the 1906 earthquake but was torn down in 1954 so that the space could be used as a parking lot. The Transamerica Pyramid, built in 1972, superseded the parking lot. Its precarious site on the shoreline necessitated a 9-foot-thick concrete and steel foundation that extends 52 feet below the sidewalk. The building has become recognized as a San Francisco icon. Note the diminishing space it occupies as it continues upward. Since the terrorist attacks on September 11, 2001, the garage and interior areas beyond the lobby have been closed to the general public.

◢ Continue right on Clay and walk past the Redwood Park (established by Transamerica for its employees and the public) to Two Transamerica Center to read the Niantic plaque. The Niantic Building, at No. 505 Sansome, was named for the abandoned ship that provided one side of the structure. The crew left for the gold mines in 1849, and the vessel was converted into a hotel. (The plaque at the location where the ship was used as a warehouse is on the Clay side of No. 505 Sansome.) Artifacts from the ship found during the excavation of the Transamerica Pyramid site are displayed on the 14th floor of Washington Towers at No. 655 Montgomery (open Monday–Friday, 9 a.m.–5 p.m.).

◢ Return to and walk through Redwood Park, which is open Monday–Friday during business hours. It is a popular place for people to bring their lunch and, during the summer, listen to noon jazz concerts. It is also a sculpture garden and has two of the best outdoor pieces in the city. The bronze *Puddle Jumpers* by Glenna Goodacre is a group of six children, whose movements—jumping rope, skipping, and hopping—are caught in mid-air and expressed with great joy and abandon. *The Frog Pond* by Richard Clopton is a group of brass frogs that exhibit the same delight in their pool.

◢ Exit the park on Washington. Turn left on Washington toward Montgomery. (On weekends go east on Clay to Sansome, and then left to Washington.) Cross Montgomery so that you can walk to your right on the odd-numbered side. Washington and Montgomery is a historic corner. At the tip of it, No. 701, is the triangular flatiron structure built in 1911. (The Registered Landmark Plaque No. 52 is on the Columbus side near the entrance.) The building has undergone several metamorphoses—from the Fugazi Bank to the Bank of Italy to headquarters of the Transamerica Corporation and, currently, the Church of Scientology.

- Continue up Montgomery, and next to No. 735 is a plaque put in place by the California Centennials Commission and the Society of California Pioneers. The plaque refers to the New York Store, a two-story wood structure that was located here. As well as selling general merchandise, the store was the receiving, sorting, and dispersal point for the first regulation mail shipment that arrived on the steamer *Oregon* in 1849. The second historic event in the store was the celebration of the Jewish New Year in September of that same year by a group of 40 Jewish pioneers who used the second floor as a synagogue. If you look up at the fire escape landings (one for each of the three floors), you will see three Stars of David on each railing that refer to this use.

- Continue on Montgomery to Jackson. The bridge that crossed Laguna Salida, the brackish inlet of Yerba Buena Cove, was located here. At No. 498, you pass the Lucas Turner & Co. Bank of 1853. General William Tecumseh Sherman, famous for his march through Georgia during the Civil War, was director of the bank for several years. A historic plaque is on the wall.

- During the Gold Rush, Jackson and Montgomery was the center of Little Chile. Chilenos, experts at using the Chilean wheel to crush gold-bearing ore, had come to work in the gold mines. (A plaque commemorating 7,000 Chilean miners is at Kearny and Columbus.)

- The Sydney Ducks, the Australian convict contingent, lived around the base of Telegraph Hill from Filbert, north, between Montgomery and Kearny. The Hounds, a group of New York toughs, lived around Grant and Pacific. The latter two groups were "hate groups," intent on eradicating people from Central and South America. Finally, after a particularly vengeful foray into Little Chile, the Vigilante group of 1851 (who called themselves the Law and Order Party) was formed under Sam Brannan's leadership to combat the plundering and marauding being carried on by the Hounds and the Ducks.

- You are in the Jackson Square Historic District, which encompasses the area from Washington to Pacific and from Columbus to Sansome.

The buildings in the 400 block of Jackson withstood the earthquake and fire of 1906, and the street has many of the earliest structures in San Francisco. Continue to the right on Jackson to Balance, the shortest street in the city. As you pass Hotaling Alley, look up at the Transamerica Pyramid. The alley was named for A. P. Hotaling's famed saloon and distillery (No. 429 Jackson). The famous two-line verse that was quoted after the quake posed a question: "If as they say God spanked the town for being over frisky / Why did he burn the churches down and save Hotaling's whiskey?"

◢ Turn left on Balance (named for the sunken ship that lies at Jackson and Front), and walk to Gold, one of the numerous alleys in this part of the city. The old three-story brick buildings are still here. (On the left is the side door of Stout Books.) Turn left on Gold and walk to Montgomery, and then turn right (north) toward Broadway. During the winter of 1849–1850, 50 inches of rain reportedly fell here. Montgomery, unpaved and unplanked, was a treacherous thoroughfare, especially at night. Wagons sank into the mud, and inebriated pedestrians had to be pulled out. An unforgettable event of that winter was the discovery of three men's bodies in the mud along Montgomery.

◢ William Stout Architectural Books at No. 804 Montgomery has one of the most complete selections in the country of books about and relating to architecture. Browsing through here is a welcome experience. The Japanesque Gallery at No. 824 Montgomery is a lovely place to stop for an aesthetically pleasing experience.

◢ Pacific Ave. illustrates so many contrasts in a few blocks. To our left where No. 549 Pacific stands (at Kearny), the scapula of a mammoth was dug up. (Hundreds of thousands of years ago, mammoths and bison roamed around here in a wet area that resembled southern Marin County.) To our right, the street is lined on both sides, predominantly with ficus trees. Behind the trees, the 19th-century, three-story brick structures contrast greatly in size with the enormous pyramid and the Bank of California. The old structures have the ambiance of a small town where you could call out the first names of all the inhabitants. At the same time, during the Gold Rush days, the section of Pacific closer to Sansome was the notorious Barbary Coast, where gangs and crime were rampant.

◢ Continue to Broadway. At the corner of Montgomery is the On-Lok organization's Senior Health Services Center, which includes 35 apartments for low-income elderly people. Seniors are brought by van and stay for the day to receive health and personal care and the midday meal. They participate in social and recreation activities and return home in the evening. One of the center's exciting programs is the ongoing, intergenerational garden shared by the elderly and about 24 children, ages two to five, from the Child Care program. With funding from several groups, including San Francisco Beautiful, the San Francisco League of Urban Gardeners, transformed the garden from an abandoned cement playground.

⊿ Turn left on Broadway, and continue to Kearny. As you ascend, you see remnants of the earlier cobblestone paving underneath your feet. Turn right to ascend the sidewalk stairway to Vallejo. At eye level you have a view of the green flatiron Zoetrope Building and the pedestrian bridge from the Hilton Hotel to Portsmouth Square.

⊿ Turn right on Vallejo. As you walk east, you come to the house at No. 448B Vallejo. It was here that Madame Luisa Tetrazzini (1871–1940), the famous Italian opera soprano, while out walking (she was on tour in San Francisco) heard the young Lina Pagliughi (born 1907) singing, when she was only 12 or 13 years old. Tetrazzini told Lina's parents she wanted to take their daughter to Italy to teach her opera and help launch her career as her successor. Lina's parents refused, but four years later, she did travel to Italy to begin her vocal studies under the direction of Tetrazzini. She subsequently had a long career with the Metropolitan Opera.

⊿ Walk down the Vallejo Stairway, designed by the Department of Public Works. The Department of Urban Forestry planted the trees and shrubs and maintains them. Neighbors have taken responsibility for additional plantings. Residents in their 70s and 80s who live adjacent to the stairway attribute their longevity to walking it daily.

⊿ Turn left on Montgomery, walk past three gingko trees, and ascend the stairway to Union. Look back to see Montgomery where it ends at Market. On a sunny day, Montgomery will be in shadow because of the high-rise buildings.

⊿ Turn right into the Union cul-de-sac. No. 291 Union, dating from 1861, is the oldest house on that block. Turn right into upper Calhoun Terrace; the Works Progress Administration built the high retaining wall that separates it in 1939. No. 9 Calhoun was built in 1854. Because it had its own spring, the owners did not request to be connected to the city water system until 1872. Walk back to Union, and turn right into lower Calhoun Terrace. No. 66 built in 1939 was designed by a Viennese architect, Richard Neutra, who espoused the International Style.

⊿ At the corner of Calhoun Terrace and Union, descend the stairway. Looking down, you will experience your elevation to Sansome St. (about 250 feet). There is no stairway down to the street because of the hazardous cliff conditions. Impatiens, century plants, snapdragons, bottlebrush, and fuchsia dot the cliff. At this site, you will likely have a good view of the wild parrots of Telegraph Hill in the cypress trees, perching and preening and teasing each other. Their cocktail hour seems to be between 4 and 5 p.m.

If you stand around and look, you can see a lot. —Yogi Berra

⊿ Ascend the stairway on the left to Union. Nos. 287, 291, and 291A were built in the 1860s. Return to Montgomery, turn right, and stop for a moment in the middle of the street to look at No. 1360. Its exterior is in the shape of a ship, complete with a shiplike upper deck. Etched into the glass over the central entrance are a gazelle, palm trees, and ocean waves. The etched panels on the side of the Art Moderne apartment house show a worker holding the world above the Bay Bridge. The real 1937 Bay Bridge towers are just beyond it. No. 1360 is also famous as the setting for the 1947 movie *Dark Passage,* which stars Humphrey Bogart and Lauren Bacall.

⊿ On your left along the retaining wall are a well-designed garden and a humorous mural featuring an apricot-colored teacup poodle named Ginger. Artists Dick Fosselman and Rick Helf cleverly incorporated the actual fire hydrant into the scene. The garden and the mural compose yet another of the surprisingly beautiful spots in this neighborhood. From here, before you descend the historic Filbert Stairway on the left side of No. 1360, you will have a better view of the etched murals.

⊿ A plaque on the Filbert Stairway expresses appreciation for Grace Marchant, who moved here in 1950, when the area was a dumping ground 30 feet deep. The city permitted her to burn the dump; it took three days to burn completely. For 30 years, Marchant labored on the stairway gardens, which were dedicated to her on May 4, 1980. She died in 1982 at the age of 96. Her neighbor, friend, and protégé, Gary Kray, cares for the gardens, and the city contributes water for their maintenance.

⊿ Darrell Place and Napier Lane are "paper streets." Although they appear as streets on maps and in street guides, Darrell is more like a

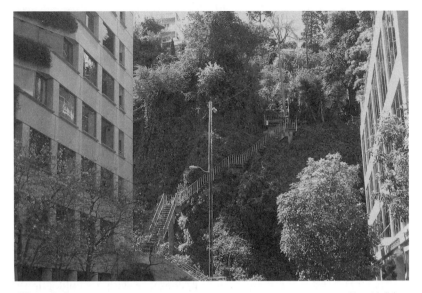

Filbert Stairway   *Tony Holiday*

trail, while Napier consists only of 12-foot wood planks. Filbert is a wood stairway threading alongside the garden. Because fire is always a hazard in these areas where there is no room for trucks, the San Francisco Fire Department stores equipment as inconspicuously as possible. Next to the blue fire hydrants on the walkway (blue is the code for connection to a high-pressure system) is a storage box for two small fire hydrants and a hose. The Gothic cottage at No. 228 (1873) was once a grocery. Next door, No. 226 is a renovated miner's shack from 1863.

◢ The lower part of Filbert Stairway is concrete. Much of the overgrown nasturtiums, fennel, and blackberries along the sides of the hill have been cut down. The design of the patterned aggregate Levi's Plaza across the street pulls us forward as we descend to Sansome. The landscaping by Lawrence Halprin Associates includes granite and trees that evoke the Sierra Nevada, where Levi Strauss began his career in 1851. Strauss supplied miners with heavy duck-cloth pants, reinforced with copper rivets, to withstand the pulling and the tearing from tools. The cloth was *serge de Nîmes* (from Nîmes, in southern France) hence, denim. If the Levi Strauss Museum is open, walk in and look around.

◢ Cross Sansome and turn right to walk on the sidewalk. As you stroll, you will become aware of the craggy east slope of Telegraph Hill, the result of years of unprofessional and unsupervised quarrying by the

Gray Bros. (1890–1903). A women's group led by Alice Griffith and Elizabeth Ashe (founders of the Telegraph Hill Neighborhood Association) enlisted support from women citywide to save Telegraph Hill from further damage. Momentum gathered, City Hall heard, and the Gray Bros.' permit was revoked.

⬧ The extraordinary plantings here now are the efforts of two neighbors who rappelled down the hill to do the work. In spring, the hillside near Green is ablaze with color from Mexican sage, primroses, poppies, *Dudleya* succulents, valerian, morning glories, tree dahlias, potato vines, and passionflower vines. *Echium* flowers grow at the edge of the hill along the street. A plaque at No. 202 Green is dedicated to Philo Farnsworth who had his laboratory there from 1926 to 1938 when he was perfecting the first functional television system. He filed more than 80 television patents.

⬧ Cross Sansome to the south corner of Green for an extraordinary view up the cliff. The back sides of three Calhoun Terrace houses supported by stilts are visible. They look as though they are imminently ready to inch forward toward Sansome.

⬧ Continue on Sansome to Broadway. Cross to One Jackson Place between Pacific and Jackson. It is a breezeway (open Monday–Friday, 8 a.m.–6 p.m.) with businesses that extend to Battery. Then walk to the corner of Battery and Jackson to get a feeling of the water geography of the mid-1800s in the city. You are now, figuratively, standing in water deep enough for the ship *Arkansas* to dock. The Old Ship Restaurant is at the location of that sunken ship where sailors were shanghaied. A plaque outside the restaurant recounts the history of the saloon. Walk on Jackson to see the name of the proprietor of that time, Henry Klee, on the top of the building. Walk back to Sansome, and then continue on toward Washington.

⬧ Turn right on Washington, and walk to Grant. At Kearny we see Portsmouth Square, the heart and outdoor living room of Chinatown, formerly the center of the Pueblo of Yerba Buena. You are dipping a toe into Chinatown, a densely populated 25-block area. It was destroyed in the 1906 earthquake but rebuilt within two years. Many of the ornate buildings were decorated in the 1920s when the community made a concerted effort to attract visitors. Grant is the tourist-oriented shopping avenue. Stockton is where the Chinese residents and knowledgeable shoppers from neighboring areas come to buy fresh produce and other food at the most reasonable prices.

On the right side of Grant, at No. 823, a plaque commemorates the first tent dwelling in Yerba Buena, which was erected in June 1835 by William Richardson, an Englishman who had deserted the English whaler *Orion* 13 years before. Industrious and helpful to the community, Richardson married the commandant's daughter and became a naturalized citizen. The plaque is on the wall on the right side of the door. If a display from the adjoining store partially covers the plaque, gently brush it aside.

There were also many hotels and theaters in this area during the 1850s: the Jenny Lind, the Phoenix, the Adelphi, and the Italian Theater, and some better-known Chinese theaters were also here.

Turn left on Grant, and walk to California. At the northeast corner is Old St. Mary's, the first Catholic cathedral in San Francisco, dedicated in 1854. It was rebuilt after being damaged in the 1906 earthquake. Still an active parish, Old St. Mary's presents a fine noon concert series and an outreach program. Turn left on California, right on Leidesdorff, and then left on Pine. Walking toward Sansome, you can see the 1930 Pacific Exchange at No. 301 Pine (now the Equinox Fitness Center) and the Ralph Stackpole sculptures flanking the entrance to the old Pacific Stock Exchange. Stackpole's quiet Art Deco giants reflect the massiveness and importance of the imposing marble building and its original purpose. Timothy Pfleuger of Miller and Pfleuger (architects) was the primary designer of the building; he was famous for the large theaters he built: the Castro and Alhambra Theatres in San Francisco and the Paramount in Oakland.

One of Adah's favorite clocks in the city is on the Furth Building at the northwest corner of Sansome. It is flanked by a lion on the left and a unicorn on the right. Let's have a look. Turn right on Sansome to walk to Market, and then turn left on Market to 1st St. and your beginning.

Further Rambling

To experience the water beneath you, walk over what once was Yerba Buena Cove. Start your walk at Commercial and Sansome in the courtyard that leads to the Embarcadero Buildings walkway. Pass the sculpture and fountain to the stairways, and ascend either one. Continue on the walkway along the One, Two, Three, and Four Embarcadero Buildings, and descend at the Embarcadero.

Old Neighborhoods

Telegraph Hill & North Beach

During the 1850s, the North Beach waterfront was a dynamic community. Conditions were in flux: there were so many people coming in, both from the eastern United States and from overseas, things were chaotic. Some were in transit, but others came to settle here. Supportive services were established—fishing boats, breweries, forges, and slaughterhouses; there were restaurants, saloons, import stores, and hostelries. People who have lived in the city for years are nostalgic about the old North Beach.

The 1906 earthquake leveled everything in this quarter except the Ferry Building, which at that time was the tallest structure in San Francisco. The area was soon rebuilt, and the city celebrated its rebirth with the Panama-Pacific International Exposition of 1915.

Over the years, the Port of San Francisco has diminished in importance. The thrust of the Port Authority's master plan is to balance maritime needs and the needs of the public. One of the plans for Fisherman's Wharf is to centralize the fish wholesalers in one facility and return the area to its original purpose—catching, preparing, and selling fish to residents and tourists alike.

WALK FACTS

Tom Cara introduced the espresso machine to the area from Italy after World War II.

Enrico Banducci introduced new entertainers, including Barbra Streisand, Woody Allen, and the Kingston Trio, at his hungry i club (for "hungry intellectual"), while comedians Lenny Bruce and Phyllis Diller first appeared at the Purple Onion, a comedy club on Columbus.

In 1990, the Court of Historical Review decided that the accordion was the official instrument of San Francisco. At one time a dozen accordion makers conducted lively businesses in North Beach.

The Beat poets held readings in the coffeehouses on upper Grant during the 1950s; Lawrence Ferlinghetti's City Lights bookstore still continues from those days (No. 261 Columbus).

The zany revue *Beach Blanket Babylon* at Club Fugazi has been performed continuously since 1974.

Bus Routes & Parking

PUBLIC TRANSPORTATION: Powell-Mason cable car; MUNI Bus #39 Coit or #30 Stockton. For MUNI bus information, call 311 (outside San Francisco, call 415-701-2311).

PARKING: There is metered street parking available; metered parking is usually for up to an hour, and free street parking is usually allowed for up to two hours. But also look for street-cleaning times posted in the

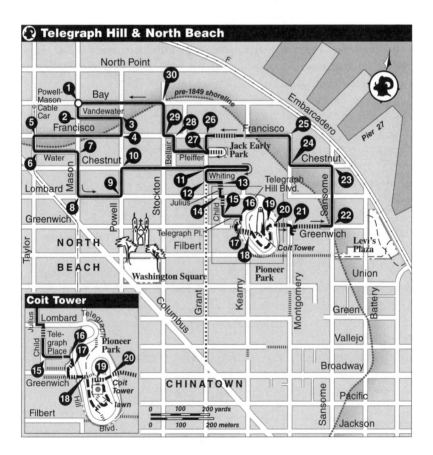

QUICK-STEP INSTRUCTIONS

1. Begin at Mason and Bay. Walk south on Mason to Vandewater.
2. Left on Vandewater to Powell.
3. Right on Powell to Francisco.
4. Right on Francisco to Taylor.
5. Left on Taylor to Water.
6. Left on Water to Mason.
7. Right on Mason to Lombard.
8. Left on Lombard to Powell.
9. Left on Powell to Chestnut.
10. Right on Chestnut past Grant to end of street. Return to Grant.
11. Left to No. 1834 Grant at Whiting.
12. Left on Whiting.
13. Midway on right, ascend Julius St. Stairway and walkway to Lombard.
14. Left to No. 383 Lombard, and ascend Child St. Stairway and walkway to Telegraph Place.
15. Left on Telegraph Place to Telegraph Hill Blvd.
16. Keep right and continue up Telegraph Hill Blvd.
17. Two doors from No. 201 descend stairway into Greenwich cul-de-sac. Walk around planted area; ascend stairway to Telegraph Hill Blvd.
18. Cross Blvd. to ascend stone stairway. Cross path to new donor stairways, and ascend to front of Coit Tower and JCDecaux toilet area.
19. Walk to the plaque designed by Michael Manwaring below stairway in front of tower. Explore area and then continue on paths around tower.
20. Go around to the front of the tower. Then bear right to cross the boulevard, and descend the Greenwich Stairway to Montgomery.
21. Cross Montgomery. Go right to lower Montgomery. Next to No. 1460, descend to continue down Greenwich Stairway.
22. Left on Sansome to Chestnut.
23. Left on Chestnut to Montgomery.
24. Right on Montgomery to Francisco.
25. Left on Francisco. Ascend stairway to Francisco cul-de-sac and Grant.
26. Left on Grant to ascend stairway to Jack Early Park on left side of street.
27. Return to Grant, and cross the street to walk through Pfeiffer St. to Bellair Place to Francisco.
28. Left on Francisco to Stockton.
29. Right on Stockton to Bay.
30. Left on Bay to Mason to your beginning.

neighborhood to avoid getting ticketed or towed. North Beach also has parking lots that charge fees.

WALK 2 DESCRIPTION

◢ You begin in a historic area of North Beach—at the intersection of Mason and Bay. During the Gold Rush days, North Beach extended only to Francisco St., near the water line. Henry "Honest Harry" Meiggs, a New York State lumberman, built a sawmill and one of the first wharfs extending into the Bay (between Mason and Powell) and established a thriving lumber trade (with imports from Oregon). At the time Fisherman's Wharf was known as Meiggs' Wharf.

◢ Genial, well-liked, and a cofounder of the San Francisco Philharmonic Society, Meiggs could charm both politicians and power brokers, and invested heavily in real estate in the North Beach area and neighborhoods farther west, believing that the area would develop rapidly. But he was wrong and found himself in the untenable position of being personally bankrupt. And, since he had embezzled City funds, he was also responsible for a financial crisis in San Francisco. Banks closed, many permanently, and investors lost their savings. In 1854, "Honest Harry" managed to sail away to Chile, where he subsequently made another fortune building a railroad through the mountains to Peru. Though he repaid most of his San Francisco debts, he died in Lima, Peru, in 1877, having been denied return to California.

◢ From the intersection of Mason and Bay, walk south on Mason. Turn left on Vandewater St. It was under water in 1849, and then in later years it evolved into a charming "twitton," as the British call it. Trees and three- and four-story apartment buildings soften the paved street.

◢ Continue to Powell, and turn right on Francisco. Until 1980, the historical site at Nos. 411–445 was the Bauer-Schweitzer Malt Company, the last barrel-malting factory west of the Mississippi. Their high-quality malt was sold to small American breweries, such as Anchor, and was also exported to Japan. When it became economically unfeasible to continue operations, the building was sold. The North Beach Malt House condominium complex is an exemplary historic conversion. Malting equipment was used imaginatively in sculptures designed for the courtyard, as well as in historical displays in the lobbies. This area is not open to the public.

◢ Turn left onto Taylor and then turn left again onto Water, another block-long twitton. It is a remnant of early San Francisco fish houses, warehouses, and bordellos. Turn right on Mason.

◢ Continue on Mason to No. 661 Lombard to view the renovated Joe DiMaggio North Beach Playground and pool. No. 660 Lombard, the Telegraph Hill Neighborhood Center, was founded in 1890 by Elizabeth Ashe and Alice Griffith to provide services to low-income immigrant families. Their efforts focused on resisting the quarrying of the hill, providing a settlement house at the crest of Vallejo for nursing care, a boys' club, and classes in homemaking and family counseling. When the newcomers realized these services were genuine, they began giving fruit and vegetables to the house, and an evening club for girls working in the canneries was begun. Griffith and Ashe were inspired by the work of Jane Addams of Chicago's Hull House, and that spirit continues today.

◢ After the 1906 earthquake, they set up a tent city in Washington Square Park and worked on legislation to prevent sleazy rebuilding. Currently, the program at the neighborhood center includes health and educational services for new immigrants from the Pacific Rim, seniors, and children of preschool age and older. Gardening is a favorite activity for all generations at the center, as evidenced by the inviting flower beds in the front and vegetable garden in the back.

◢ One of the most abundant displays of cascading, fuchsia-colored bougainvillea in the city adorns No. 604 Lombard. The vine was planted in 1938; it blooms twice a year, and each year it becomes more exuberant. Its color contrasts beautifully with the six junipers (whose shapes suggest ladybugs) planted along the wall of the apartment house.

◢ Turn left on Powell and right on Chestnut. Continue walking two blocks to Grant and Chestnut. No. 298 Chestnut is a Mediterranean-style home built in 1929. Its tile roof, marble entry, and ceramic Della Robbia plaque are visible through the iron gates. Walk to the end of the Kearny cul-de-sac along the left side (designated as "open space") to obtain a view of the "lowlands."

◢ Here you have a long view of Marin County toward the north and west. Besides the boats anchored at Pier 39, you can see Piers 33 and 35 and perhaps a container ship proceeding toward the Port of Oakland. Pier 39 is well known for its fine horticultural displays of container flowers, a colony of sea lions that has taken up residence along the wharf, good restaurants, and friendly stores. The outdoor spaces encourage strolling, and the area is very popular with young people and children. It's also a great place to watch fireworks on the Fourth of July. (These reasons balance out the architecture.) Angel Island State Park is visible to the north.

⊿ Return to Grant. At Grant turn left (south) and left again into Whiting cul-de-sac. Three-fourths of the way down the block and to the right, ascend the nine steps of Julius St. Stairway, and walk to the end, which brings you to Lombard. Across the street to the left of No. 383 is the short Child St. Stairway.

⊿ Walk up to Telegraph Place, and continue to Telegraph Hill Blvd. Turn right. Next to No. 201, descend a stairway into the Greenwich St. cul-de-sac. Circle the planted oval area dedicated to Maria Pimentell for her 25 years of gardening. Walk up the opposite stairway to Telegraph Hill Blvd.

⊿ Cross the boulevard to ascend the stone stairway leading to the footpath. Cross the footpath and ascend the stairway with donors' names to the top. In the early days, it was known as Signal Hill because the arrival of ships would be signaled from here across the city. In the 1880s, a restaurant was the chief attraction on the hill.

⊿ At the top, walk to the wall plaque designed by Michael Manwaring. It notes the historical timetable of the Pioneer Park Project surrounding Coit Tower. Arthur Brow Jr.'s original landscape plan for the area surrounding the 1933 Coit Tower, which he also designed, was finally completed in 2002. Fulfilling a historic mission to bring beauty to it for all to share, the park also emphasizes contemporary history, as its stairs carry the inscriptions of the names of people who contributed to its fundraising.

⊿ Lillie Hitchcock Coit, who had fond memories from childhood when she was a mascot for Knickerbocker Engine Company No. 5, one of the city's volunteer firefighting companies, funded the construction of Coit Tower, which was dedicated in 1933. The tower rises 179 feet from the crest of Telegraph Hill, itself 284 feet high.

⊿ Walk to the footpath on your right, where you will see an excellent map of San Francisco on the side of the JCDecaux public toilet. Continue to Pioneer Park, at the back of Coit Tower. There are low retaining walls where you can sit, have your lunch, and enjoy the views of eastern, southern, and western San Francisco. On sunny days, many people come to Coit Tower to eat their lunch, enjoy the conviviality, and return to work refreshed.

◢ The Pioneer Park Project began as a dedicated, determined, and formidable pro bono grassroots group of volunteers who worked for six years to raise the money for the construction of three new stairways leading to Coit Tower, a picnic area overlooking the Bay, a wheelchair-accessible ramp, and the planting of native plants and trees. This large-scale beautification undertaking is one of the finest examples of commitment, intelligent planning, and consistent involvement by Telegraph Hill neighbors, as well as the cooperation of the City of San Francisco and other interested residents. The project matches in scale

Telegraph Hill, ca. 1880

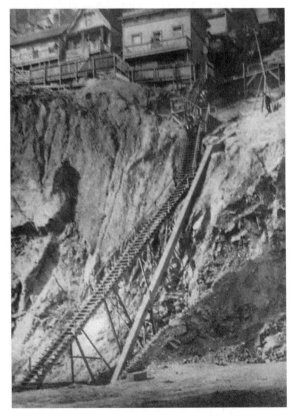

the 1876 purchase of the four lots at the crest of Telegraph Hill by San Francisco citizens, who subsequently transferred ownership to the city.

◢ The view to the east of the graceful 1895 Ferry Building and its famous clock is distinctive. (Lit up at night, it is a cameo, a Cinderella, surpassing all other commercial buildings in its delicate beauty.)

◢ The tall, slender Embarcadero buildings to the southeast are on the site of the old wholesale produce market. Because Embarcadero Center is on redevelopment land and federal funds partially defrayed building costs, the developer was obliged to spend 1% of the total project cost on artwork. The result is that excellent sculpture is located throughout the center. Directly in front of you is the Transamerica Pyramid, built on the original shoreline (Walk 1). The 48-story dark carnelian granite structure is the Bank of America Building on California.

◢ As you walk along the right side of Coit Tower, look inside and see the Works Progress Administration murals executed in the 1930s. Intermittent vandalism and damage from water seepage have necessitated closing the mural rooms to visitors from time to time. The elevator ride to the top floor is available to the public at a nominal charge. The parking lot has coin telescopes to bring Marin County and the East Bay into close-up view.

◢ Walk down the front stairs of the tower, take the footpath to the right, and cross Telegraph Hill Blvd. to descend the Greenwich Stairway. The upper brick section of the stairway curves, allowing room on each side for wide, terraced, private gardens. The unnamed lane running at a right angle from No. 356 Greenwich connects with the Filbert Stairway farther south (Walk 1).

◢ The first landing of these 147 stairs leads down to the Montgomery cul-de-sac and the now closed Landmark 121 Julius Castle restaurant, built in 1923. A beautiful, mature fig tree graces the entrance. Because the lower retaining wall was designed in a random pattern of brick with protruding stones, which is extremely photogenic, look back before you descend the next set of stairs.

◢ Cross Montgomery (you may feel like an opera singer taking a deep breath), and bear right to the Greenwich sign. Descend the concrete stairs and extended walkways. Along the way you see a cistern for firefighting, and, on the left side of the walkway, trees (a magnificent magnolia) and gardens (roses and irises, as well as ferns and fuchsias).

The resident flock of wild parrots hangs out here and obtains sustenance from juniper berries and loquats near No. 243 Greenwich.

◢ Mark Bittner, who lives nearby, was able to watch the parrots from a vantage point where he did not frighten them. He observed them over a period of years, and they learned to trust him, eat from his hand, and sit on his shoulder. When he began observing and feeding them, there were 25 in the flock. He says there are between 180 and 200 birds living on the hill. Bittner learned their behavior patterns and their individual quirks, named them, and fed the flock for several years. He no longer feeds them because he says the parrots are finding enough food to eat on their own. They have been seen in Glen Park, Fort Mason, and Russian Hill, and they roost in Walton Square. The highly acclaimed documentary film *The Wild Parrots of Telegraph Hill* by Judy Irving has been seen throughout the United States and Europe. Bittner's book is a beautifully told story about how his life has been affected by the parrots, by Irving, and by his writing. In June 2006, Bittner and Irving were married, and Telegraph Hill celebrated.

◢ The Parks, Trees, and Birds Committee of the Telegraph Hill Dwellers, under Irving's leadership, has taken on the responsibility of clearing overgrowth and invasive plants in the area. Hired professional arborists are removing dead wood and pruning the healthy trees. In clearing out and cutting back the ivy, they discovered a California coast live oak. It has several trunks and is probably 50 to 60 years old. There are 15 varieties of trees in the canyon. Valetta Hazlett, daughter of Grace Marchant (see Walk 1), planted the Deodar cedars that grow here more than 60 years ago. Along the footpath of the canyon, resident artists have randomly placed pieces of sculpture and mosaics and whimsical items, like the parking meter in back of the comfortable bench. These constantly change, but what a delight for residents and visitors to be alerted to these favors. On certain days, you may find yourself surrounded by hummingbirds. At the foot of the steps, turn left on Sansome and continue north.

◢ The slope of Telegraph Hill, now barely visible from Sansome and Lombard since the Lombard Plaza apartments were built in 1991, was the amphitheater for a 1966 Janis Joplin rock concert.

◢ Turn left on Chestnut. A three-story brick structure (originally built in the late 1800s and reconstructed in 1973) is angled across the corner of Montgomery. You turn right on Montgomery and left on Francisco.

◢ At the cross street of Kearny, walk into the well-cared-for courtyard of the Wharf Plaza, a subsidized housing complex for seniors and families. The gardens are a pleasant place for the residents to sit and visit, and in September the area is spectacular with gingko trees ringed in gold leaves. Ascend the well-designed stairway. It features an unusual, long, elevated walkway—perfect for a stairway dance performance. At the top of the stairway, you reach the Francisco cul-de-sac. The Telegraph Terrace condos fit snugly into the block and around the corner onto Grant.

Phyllis Pearsall (1906–1996), the founder of Geographer's A–Z Map Company, walked for 18 hours (beginning at 5 a.m.) daily, to list a total of 23,000 roads in London. Asked if she got lost in London, she replied, "Always, dear." During her lifetime, she walked 3,000 miles.

◢ Turn left on Grant. In the middle of the block, make another left to walk up the stairs to Jack Early Park. Beginning in 1962 Jack Early ("Mr. Tree"), in a one-man effort, started planting trees and flowers in a neglected area. When Adah spoke to him, he remembered carrying water buckets by hand from his house on Pfeiffer. Now maintained by the Telegraph Terrace Association, the park is a rewarding place for views, solitude, and moon-watching.

◢ Come back down the stairway, cross Grant, and walk through Pfeiffer Alley, a right-of-way that has become a special enclave. Nos. 139–141 date from 1910, and No. 152 from 1891.

◢ Turn right into Bellair Place. Paving stones and recessed spaces for plants are welcoming tokens of promise. Make a left on Francisco, and cross the street to see the little cottage at No. 276, which dates from 1863. Delicious aromas emanate from No. 271, Tante Marie's Cooking School.

◢ Continue west on Francisco to Stockton. Turn right to Bay, and left to the beginning of the walk.

Further Rambling

By now you have explored some of the twittons, lanes, alleyways, and right-of-ways that are plentiful here in North Beach. If you would like to explore the neighborhood shopping areas on Columbus or upper Grant, you will find lots of foot traffic, small shops, restaurants, and coffeehouses with outdoor tables and chairs. Many old, Italian businesses have closed; Chinese signs are now more common on stores.

Washington Square, the piazza on Stockton between Union and Filbert (now City Landmark No. 226), was reserved as a park in the city plan of 1847 and sheltered some of the 1906 earthquake homeless in prefabricated camp cottages. Fragments of memories that people have shared over the years compose the ambiance of North Beach. First-time visitors may not share this background, but the abundance of specialty stores at street level, the number of eating and drinking establishments, general friendliness, and the density of neighborhood foot traffic all invite further exploring.

To connect to Walk 6, follow Mason to Bay and then head west. You can begin Walk 2 near the Safeway at Laguna and the Great Meadow.

Castles in the Air

Nob Hill

Nob Hill, 376 feet above the Bay, is wedged between Pacific Heights to the west, Russian Hill to the north, and North Beach and Chinatown to the east. Millions of tourists have traversed Nob Hill on the cable cars, gliding both north–south on Powell between Market and Fisherman's Wharf and east–west on California. The Powell line began operations in 1887; the California St. cable railway began in 1878.

A paradox of this walk is that its most interesting characteristics can be noted by standing still and looking up to make out the lofty architectural details on the buildings, while also registering the delight of cable car riders at eye level. Binoculars add extended range to your sightings.

Nob Hill is famous for its views, luxury hotels, and apartment houses. The only "neighbors" in this section may be doormen, hotel guests alighting from a taxi, or the elderly rich assisted by nurses or companions. But there is a neighborhood, and in the side streets and alleyways, there are neighbors to visit and talk to, and who might even share garden cuttings. The Nob Hill Association, the neighborhood watchdog organization founded in 1923, is actively concerned with the environment and community issues.

When you think historically about Victorian life on Nob Hill, you can't help but think about the extravagance and lavish tastes and wants of the wives of the Big Four—Jane Stanford, Arabella Huntington, Elizabeth Hopkins, and Mary Ann Crocker. While their husbands were making decisions in their offices on how to amass millions, these ladies were making decisions in their corporate headquarters (the interiors of their mansions) on how to outdo each other by the millions. Imagine them contemplating, "Should I use mahogany for the cabinets, or should I wait for the ship from Africa to bring in teak and rosewood? Should I buy that Michelangelo, or should I have someone copy it?" Conspicuous consumption merrily reigned. Only Elizabeth Hopkins may have had any issues, since lavishness was the opposite of her husband's frugality, his vegetarianism, and his dislike of the ornate furniture she bought. It's difficult to imagine how the wives might have fared if they had come west on the Oregon and California Trails via covered wagon.

WALK FACTS

Grace Cathedral honors St. Francis and his love of animals each year in October by blessing pets on a special day.

The Tonga Room still offers a floating band and a scheduled typhoon (every 20 minutes or so) in the old Olympic Pool at the Fairmont Hotel. It may seem touristy, but it's one of the most San Francisco things you can do, so why not enjoy a snack, a cocktail, and an indoor rainstorm?

Bus Routes & Parking

PUBLIC TRANSPORTATION: California St. Cable Car; MUNI Bus #27 Bryant and #1 California. For MUNI bus information, call 311 (outside San Francisco, call 415-701-2311).

PARKING: There is metered street parking available; metered parking is usually available for up to an hour, and free street parking is usually allowed for up to two hours. But also look for street-cleaning times posted in the neighborhood to avoid getting ticketed or towed. There is also paid, pubic parking available at the Nob Hill Masonic Center at California and Jones.

WALK 3 DESCRIPTION

⊿ Begin at California and Leavenworth on the crest of Nob Hill. Walk north on Leavenworth, along the odd-numbered side for a few yards, and turn left into Acorn Alley. Usually it is full of plants and color during the growing season.

⊿ From Acorn, turn left on Leavenworth toward Sacramento. Dashiell Hammett lived in the brick and stucco building on the corner at No. 1155 while he finished writing *The Maltese Falcon.* Chico's grocery store at No. 1168 Leavenworth was a neighborhood legend when it was in the Chico family from 1929 to 1997. (No longer owned by the family, it is still run as a grocery store with the same name.) Any long-time Nob Hill resident can tell you tales of the special favors the

QUICK-STEP INSTRUCTIONS

1. Begin at California and Leavenworth. Walk north on Leavenworth to Acorn Alley.
2. Left on Acorn. Return to Leavenworth.
3. Left on Leavenworth to Clay.
4. Return to Sacramento. Left on Sacramento to Golden Court.
5. Right on Golden. Return to Sacramento.
6. Right on Sacramento to Leroy Place.
7. Right on Leroy. Return to Sacramento.
8. Left on Leroy. Return to Sacramento.
9. Left on Sacramento to Jones.
10. Left on Jones to Pleasant.
11. Right on Pleasant to Taylor.
12. Right on Taylor to Sacramento.
13. Left on Sacramento to Powell.

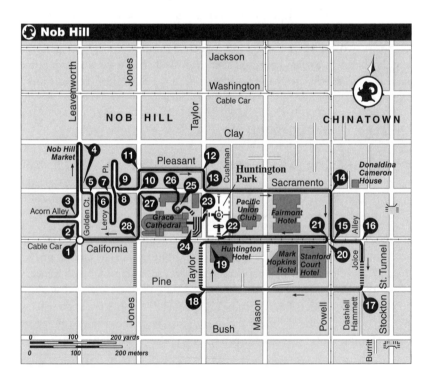

14. Right on Powell to California.

15. Left on California to Joice Alley.

16. Right on Joice. Descend stairway to Pine.

17. Right on Pine to Taylor.

18. Right on Taylor Stairway to California.

19. Right on California to Powell.

20. Left on Powell.

21. Left on California past Cushman.

22. Ascend stairway into Huntington Park.

23. Descend stairway from the park at Taylor.

24. Cross Taylor. Ascend stairway to Grace Cathedral to explore the interior, labyrinth, and courtyard.

25. Follow walkway across from fountain in the courtyard to Sacramento.

26. Left on Sacramento to Jones.

27. Left on Jones to California.

28. Right on California to your beginning.

two brothers, then later their sons (cousins) did for their customers. Their grocery was a Nob Hill institution. When neighbors went on vacation, they left their keys with them. Chico's always had access to their apartments to deliver groceries. When customers ordered items they did not stock, the grocers secured it elsewhere. In emergencies, they used their truck to drive someone to the hospital or doctor.

When Louis Montesquieu (born in 1689) arrived in a new town, he liked to climb up a high tower to get a good overall look at the place and then come down and examine the different parts at leisure.

Cross Sacramento to see the corner building with two addresses, Nos. 1202–1206 Leavenworth and Nos. 1380–1390 Sacramento. Designed by Julia Morgan in 1910, it is a Craftsman-style shingle structure. Morgan worked in the San Francisco Bay Area from about 1905 to the 1930s, designing Craftsman-style homes and also elegant structures, such as the Hearst Castle in San Simeon, California.

Continue on Leavenworth to No. 1263, Nob Hill Market (known as Le Beau), an inviting grocery, deli, and bakery that has been in this location for more than two decades. High-quality produce, fish, and other meats are available. Their take-out sandwiches complement a walk nicely. The mural on the Leavenworth side and another on the Clay side, plus changing art exhibits within the store, attest to the owner's interests and the conviviality of the ambiance.

◢ Return to Sacramento, turn left, and walk on the odd-numbered side. The foliage of evenly spaced ficus street trees adds a softness that makes this section of Sacramento inviting.

◢ Turn right into Golden Court. The name *Golden* is on the upper side of the first house. Shrubs of yellow, white, and orange datura are planted on both sides of the walkway. The owner built the gray asbestos-sided house on our right in 1950 (the address is officially No. 1154 Leavenworth) on the only empty lot on the street. He planted the *tiglio* (known in the United States as the linden) tree in 1947 from a seedling his mother brought in her purse from Italy. Golden Court is especially photogenic.

◢ Leroy Place, our next right turn off Sacramento, has two symmetrical rows of ficus trees that frame the walk and cul-de-sac. No. 16 Leroy has attractive bowed windows. Go across Sacramento into the continuation of Leroy. Tall bottlebrush trees on one side and ficus trees on the other enhance the short alley. A basilica-shaped structure at the end of the street is the back of No. 1239 Jones, the Tank High Pressure System of the San Francisco Fire Department.

◢ Walk out of the cul-de-sac, and make a left turn on Sacramento. No. 1315–1325 is a six-flat Edwardian. Continue to Jones.

◢ Grace Episcopal Cathedral School for Boys is on the lower level of the corner of the square block that includes the diocesan house and the cathedral itself. You can see its brightly colored playground equipment. The school was built in 1966 for children from kindergarten through eighth grade. Turn left on Jones.

◢ The 1200 and 1300 blocks feature luxury apartments and restaurants: No. 1221 Jones, No. 1250, and the Comstock Apartments at No. 1333. Next to No. 1234, turn right into Pleasant. *Metrosideros* trees line the sidewalk. No. 75 Pleasant has extravagantly large north-facing windows. Across the street is the back of a concrete parking garage. A brass plate on the door of No. 40–44 admonishes, "No Smoking."

◢ Make a right turn on Taylor. Across the street at No. 1110 is the smallest structure on the block, a one-story, modified, three-window bay, originally built by James Flood, of the Comstock silver mines, for his coachman.

◢ Turn left on Sacramento. No. 1182 has a mailbox at about sidewalk level and a plaque next to it commemorating its Nob Hill architectural award for excellence in 1960. In the sidewalk to the right of No. 1182 Sacramento is a survey monument with the precise latitude and longitude of this spot inscribed under its cover.

◢ Continue east on Sacramento to Powell. You can see cars crossing the Bay Bridge through the narrow opening between skyscrapers. No. 1000 Mason is the elegant Brocklebank Apartments, built in 1924. Ornate mythological beasts are positioned atop the entrance. (Hitchcock's *Vertigo* was filmed here.)

◢ Turn right at Powell to California. The left side of the street is lined with apartments. You can see the octagonal green-and-white, electronically operated traffic control tower for the cable car system at California and Powell.

◢ Turn left on California to Joice. Ahead at No. 845 is a pleasingly symmetrical Art Deco apartment house with a marble entrance and elaborate light fixtures. Turn right on Joice to the stairway and descend. Two magnolia trees are planted at the first landing. A small shrine to St. Francis is on the lower landing near the graceful curve of the stairs at Pine. The flats, Nos. 738, 740, and 742 Pine are built in the Pueblo style. Across the street is what was once known as Monroe Alley, but is now Dashiell Hammett St. His fans may want to detour over to Bush and go into Burritt Alley (between Stockton and Powell) to read the bronze plaque about his novel *The Maltese Falcon.*

◢ Turn right on Pine. At the corner, above the high parapet on the rear of the Stanford Court Hotel, is a cast-stone penguin by Beniamino "Benny" Bufano, the impecunious artist and bohemian who captured the imagination of San Franciscans and, more importantly, the financial support of patrons in the mid-20th century. At the time of his death in 1970, many of his works were stored in warehouses. Others are scattered in several places: in the courtyard of the California Academy of Sciences, at the Phelan St. entrance to the science building of San Francisco City College, in the meadow at Fort Mason (Walk 6), on the grounds of the low-cost housing at 370 Valencia, and in the Ordway Building lobby in Oakland.

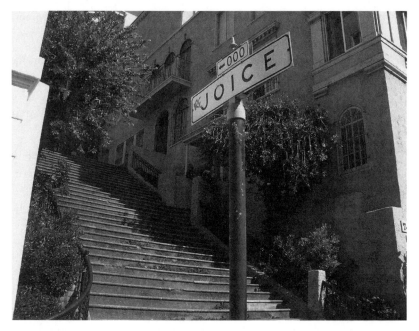

Joice Stairway   *Tony Holiday*

⌐ On Pine, you are now walking along the route of the original granite
retaining wall of the Leland Stanford mansion, which was destroyed
by the earthquake. The blocked entrance in the wall may have been
for tradesmen. The tower with the finial marks the division between
the properties of two of the Big Four railroad barons, Stanford and
Mark Hopkins. The wall surrounds these properties from Pine to
California and Powell to Mason.

⌐ Turn right on Taylor, and ascend the sidewalk stairway to California.
As your bird's-eye view from the top—California between Taylor and
Powell—comes into focus, you see lines of formidable structures: the
Fairmont, Mark Hopkins, and Huntington Hotels and the Pacific
Union Club. The Stanford Court Hotel anchors the Powell side; Grace
Cathedral and the Cathedral Apartments are on the Jones side. The
secondary line along Sacramento consists of luxury apartments.

⌐ Turn right on California to the Big Four Restaurant, at No. 1075, in
the Huntington Hotel, considered by many people to be one of the
city's most elegant hotels. You are welcome to come in between 4 and
5:30 p.m. to view the panoramic photograph of 1878 San Francisco
by Eadweard Muybridge. It is located at the end of the restaurant, to
your right.

◢ Continuing on California, we come to No. 1021. Ornate wrought iron double doors provide the entrance to this single-family dwelling; French doors are on the second story. Another notable structure is No. 1001, the Morsehead apartment building (constructed in 1915). Behind the terra-cotta columns and facade are eight apartments, each between 2,000 and 3,000 square feet. The building feels cozier than many on the block.

◢ Cross Mason to No. 999 California, the Mark Hopkins Hotel, originally the site of his home. The hotel opened in 1925. Across Mason, opposite the car entry of the hotel, is a graduated series of town houses, Nos. 831–849 Mason. Designed by Willis Polk around 1918, they provide an imaginative counterfoil to the sumptuous structures on the hill.

◢ Turn right and walk down California. Plaques on the side of the Mark Hopkins wall recount some of the site's history. Continue to No. 905, the Stanford Court Hotel, built in 1911. The glass dome sits above the Aurea restaurant next to the hotel's registration area.

◢ Continue on California to Powell. Cross Powell and turn left on California. Walk up to Mason to the white granite Fairmont Hotel, at No. 950, which was readied for its grand opening in 1906. On April 18 at 5:15 a.m., the fire caused by the earthquake destroyed the interior. Luckily, the fire insurance didn't expire until midnight! The steel frame survived, and a year later, the hotel opened for business. A contemporary feature of the Fairmont is its exterior elevator, which provides an unusual kinetic experience as you gradually ascend while watching the cityscape.

◢ As you walk along California, you will see to the right No. 1000, the landmark Pacific Union Club, a private social club with membership by invitation only. James Flood built this brownstone building as his residence in 1886. It is the only one of the mansions on Nob Hill to have survived the fire of 1906 because it was the only one not built of wood. Willis Polk reconstructed and remodeled the home in 1912. The legend that has trickled down through the generations (which we all like to believe, not much caring if it's fact or fiction) says that Flood hired a full-time maintenance man to keep the bronze fence around the property polished.

◢ Continue on California past Cushman to ascend the stairway into Huntington Park. Arabella, the widow of Collis P. Huntington, one of the Big Four railroad barons, donated Huntington Park across the street to the city in 1915. The Huntington home on the property was demolished by the 1906 quake. The park is well designed for both adults and children. The northern section has swings, slides, and a large sandbox. The middle and southern section features the Fountain of the Turtles, a delight to contemplate while sitting on the comfortable bench. The Nob Hill Association, in conjunction with Friends of Recreation and Parks, financed a recent renovation of the park and has undertaken the responsibility for maintaining it. Descend the stairway from the park at Taylor, and cross the street.

⬛ You are now on the block where Charles Crocker, one of the Big Four railroad kings, built his home. Crocker wanted to own the entire square block. Angered by the audacity of his neighbor who refused to sell his lot at a reasonable price, Crocker built a 40-foot-tall "spite fence" that cut off the sun and view from three sides of Nicholas Yung's home at No. 1203 Sacramento. But Yung, the German mortician who would not sell his property to Crocker, was undaunted. Yung retaliated by putting a curse on Crocker's life, when he built a 10-foot long coffin with a skull and crossbones and positioned it on his roof to face Crocker's house. How did Mary Ann Crocker feel about the spite fence or the skull and crossbones? It is not clear. The 1906 fire demolished both structures, and both men eventually died. Only then were the Crocker heirs able to buy the Yung property from his estate. The Crocker estate later donated the land to the diocese on which the Grace Cathedral complex is now located.

⬛ Ascend the Grand Stairway to the cathedral that leads you to the magnificent, cast-bronze doors made from the molds of the Renaissance sculptor Lorenzo Ghiberti. High above the doors, you face the rose-window facade of Grace Cathedral.

⬛ Traditionally, cathedrals are built over a period of many years. Grace Cathedral is true to this tradition. The cornerstone of Grace Cathedral was laid in 1910; the exterior was completed in 1964; in 1993, an $11 million construction project completed the design as envisioned by the original architect, Lewis Hobart, who was inspired by Notre Dame. Samuel Yellin executed the subdued, elegant wrought ironwork on the gates to the Chapel of Grace, on the south side nearest the California St. entrance. Murals by Antonio Sotomayor, chronicling cathedral and parish history, are inside the chapel. (For a better appreciation of the items in the interior, use one of the self-guided tour pamphlets available at the entrance.)

⬛ Concerts—sacred, secular, organ, choral, or jazz—are regularly presented. Acoustics are excellent, with a 7- to 12-second delay, depending on the pitch of the instrument. Duke Ellington was commissioned by the diocese to compose a sacred piece, which was performed at a concert in 1965. During the Christmas season of 1990, Bobby McFerrin, the San Francisco singer and conductor, organized a 24-hour sing-a-thon "healing," with various musical groups participating.

◢ To the right of the Grand Stairway is a labyrinth, based on the one at Chartres Cathedral, a tool for meditative walking. Ascend the Bishop Pike Stairway to a wide courtyard, fountain, and cloister. All of these are named for the donors. The Gothic trefoil design repeated on the stained glass windows and the fountain subtlety unites these parts of the grand cathedral complex. Across from the fountain, walk through the cloister to Sacramento.

◢ Turn left on Sacramento to Jones and left on Jones. From here, looking south, you can see the San Bruno Mountains. At California, near Jones, are a cluster of large apartment and condo buildings—the 1200 Corporation at No. 1200 California, the Cathedral Apartments at No. 1201 California, and the Gramercy Towers condominiums at 1177 California (next to the Masonic Auditorium).

◢ Turn right on California to Leavenworth to your beginning.

Further Rambling

Two blocks before the beginning of this walk, look for the Donaldina Cameron House at No. 920 Sacramento, which was formerly the Chinese Presbyterian Mission Home. The mission began efforts in 1874 to rescue young Chinese girls brought to San Francisco as factory slaves and prostitutes. Donaldina Cameron joined the group in 1895 and continued her missionary work for 40 years. The house currently provides community recreational and social services. The clinker-brick structure was built in 1881 and then rebuilt in 1907 by Julia Morgan.

The Nob Hill walk is very close to Walks 1, 2, and 7. Each of these walks packs a lot of history and culture into a very small amount of space, with a lot of good stairways too. Plus if the weather is good or bad, shopping is a constant distraction as you stroll among the hills downtown and to the Bay. Pace yourself, and take time to appreciate the views and tiny surprises you'll find along the way. Maybe even try going half your regular pace and see what catches your eye.

$\int$peaking of $\int$ntangibles

Russian Hill South

Every San Francisco neighborhood has its unique ambiance, a distillation of the folklore and stories of its early days surviving through continual modifications. Russian Hill acquired its name from an early cemetery located on the east side of Vallejo and Jones where Russian sailors were buried before the Gold Rush (a stairway is located on the site). Greek Orthodox crosses and bones have been unearthed there. The sailors had probably come down from Fort Ross, the Russian settlement, with the pelts of seals and otters.

In the late 1800s and even more so after the 1906 earthquake demolished other structures, small cottages expressing the special ambiance of the neighborhood adorned Russian Hill. The active Russian Hill Neighbors Association is working diligently to preserve this sense of neighborhood in the face of great economic and demographic changes. They have fought the demolition of cottages and their replacement with three- and four-story condominiums. Only about 38 cottages remain out of the 100 originally built.

Russian Hill is a craggy, physically compact area. Jasper O'Farrell, the City surveyor, extended the street grid to Leavenworth in 1847. Somehow, working theoretically and on paper, he didn't make allowance for the hills. As a result of the rectangular street configuration, the summit of Russian Hill became isolated. At Jones a ladder was placed against the bluff to access the 1000 block of Vallejo. Broadway, Vallejo, and Green were impassable for horse teams. These features attracted people who desired a measure of independence with proximity to the city center. The hilltop housing sites made possible the magnificent views, which are still a reason to live on Russian Hill. The topography also encouraged a sense of community among residents. For many years, a large coterie of writers, including Bret Harte, George Sterling, and Ina Coolbrith, resided on the hill.

WALK FACTS

Between Jones and Leavenworth on Green St., one of two surviving octagonal houses built in San Francisco still stands, having survived the 1906 earthquake and fire. This private residence was built in 1858, according to plans popularized by the perfection movement of individuals and self that sprang up in the mid-19th century. Phrenologist Orson Squire Fowler lectured that octagonal houses were warmer and cheaper to build.

Before or after your walk, hop on a cable car, and take a ride on the running boards (but do hold on). The Powell-Hyde and Powell-Mason cable car lines both run through this walk.

Bus Routes & Parking

PUBLIC TRANSPORTATION: MUNI Bus #19 Polk; #47 and #49 Van Ness. For MUNI bus information, call 311 (outside San Francisco call 415-701-2311).

PARKING: There is metered street parking available; metered parking is usually available for up to an hour, and free street parking is usually allowed for up to two hours. But also look for street-cleaning times posted in the neighborhood to avoid getting ticketed or towed.

WALK 4 DESCRIPTION

▗ Begin at the northeast corner of Polk and Greenwich, where Russian Hill begins its sharp rise toward Larkin. Walk up a partially grooved sidewalk. No. 1342–1344 is a relatively new condominium. The garage has been embellished with a band of decorative ceramic tile placed above its doors.

▗ Turn right on Larkin to Filbert, and then left. The 1200 block of Filbert, from Larkin to Hyde, is composed mostly of Edwardian flats with bay windows on the two upper stories. The block has few trees, but next to No. 1252 is a terraced rock garden. The angled stairway at No. 1234 with its landings appears like a hopscotch diagram. The brown-shingled building at the corner, No. 1205, is designed in the Craftsman style.

QUICK-STEP INSTRUCTIONS

1. Begin at Polk and Greenwich.
2. Right on Larkin to Filbert.
3. Left on Filbert. Descend sidewalk stairway to Leavenworth.
4. Right on Leavenworth. Ascend Havens Stairway and return to Leavenworth. Turn right.
5. Left on Union to Jones.
6. Right to Macondray Lane. Left to explore and return. Right to Union. Right to Taylor.
7. Right to Green.
8. Ascend Green Stairway to Jones.
9. Left on Jones to Vallejo.
10. Left onto Vallejo Stairway into cul-de-sac, and walk to end.
11. Descend Vallejo Stairway next to No. 1019, past Taylor to Mason.

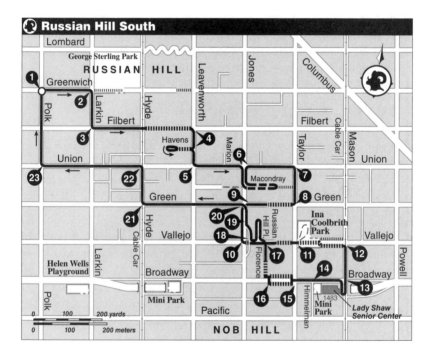

12. Right on Mason. Cross Broadway to see Lady Shaw Senior Center at No. 1483 Mason.

13. Cross back to Broadway; left (west) on Broadway.

14. Continue on Broadway past Himmelman Place Mini Park.

15. Continue west on sidewalk stairway past Taylor to Florence.

16. Ascend Florence Stairway.

17. Walk across Vallejo into Russian Hill Place.

18. Right to walk down ramp to Jones.

19. Right on Jones to Green.

20. Left on Green to Hyde.

21. Right on Hyde to Union.

22. Left on Union to Polk.

23. Right on Polk to Greenwich to your beginning

Continue past the hum of cables in the slot of Hyde to walk down the Filbert Stairway. At the bottom of the hill, turn right on Leavenworth. In a half block, next to 2033 Leavenworth, ascend Havens Stairway, a little-known stairway that can only be accessed from Leavenworth (it formerly continued through to Hyde).

The property owners living on Havens cultivate the gardens alongside the stairway. The fern garden is one of the most attractive additions to the green space. Return to Leavenworth.

At Leavenworth turn right to Union and then left. Continue to Jones and turn right. Walk into Macondray Lane through a trellised entry into an unexpected garden path, the magical part of Macondray. You see goldfish ponds, garden ornaments, and both annual and perennial plantings. The bordering condos are small but attractive. The area feels as though it ought to be private gardens, but Macondray Lane, named for a 19th-century merchant and viticulturist, is a public right-of-way. It is the setting for Armistead Maupin's *Tales of the City,* a television miniseries based on his book of the same name. The variety of trees and shrubs in every shade of green adds to its appeal.

Turn back at the cobblestone section. The footing ahead is not safe enough for walkers to continue; instead return to Jones.

⊿ Turn right on Jones. Walk to Union, and turn right. You will pass a private cul-de-sac alleyway—Marion Place. The plaque gives some of its little-known history. Turn right on Taylor and walk to Green. Ascend the stairway on the right to the cul-de-sac, passing an elaborate Art Moderne apartment house on the left, and continue on Green to see an inviting wood-frame house from the 1890s, next to No. 980.

⊿ Towering above everything in sight is No. 999 Green, the Eichler Summit Apartments, built before the height-limitation law was passed in 1970. In the center of the tower, three, long, open, oval shapes that resemble huge exclamation points appear to punctuate the end of a special block, the 1000 block of Green that escaped fire and earthquake damage in 1906.

⊿ Walk to Jones and turn left to enter the arched, double-stairway entrance to a very special section of Vallejo. It is part of Russian Hill's Vallejo St. Crest District, which is on the National Register of Historic Places. You might call this the Livermore section of Vallejo. From 1897 until 2003, some member of the family lived continuously in this enclave, staunchly supporting efforts to preserve and maintain the unique character and beauty of the area. You might also call it the Livermore and Polk section. The architect Willis Polk was hired by Horatio Livermore (and later by his son Norman) to build many of the houses and design both the entrance on Jones and the stairway to Taylor.

⊿ Continue to the end of the cul-de-sac, walking on the odd-numbered south side. No. 1023 is the Horatio Livermore house, built by Julia Morgan in 1917. A developer demolished three redwood-shingled houses at No. 1030, designed by Joseph Worcester circa 1889. They have since been replaced by the Hermitage condominium apartments, which duplicate the Craftsman style so appropriate for the nooks and crannies of Russian Hill. The architects Joseph Worcester, Julia Morgan, Bernard Maybeck, Willis Polk, and Ernest Coxhead built homes in this style during the first quarter of the 20th century as an antidote to the excesses and formalism of Victorian architecture. They emphasized natural elements: redwood shingles and protruding eaves instead of bracketed cornices and gabled roofs. Trees and shrubs were an important part of the design, and homes were designed to blend harmoniously with the topography.

⊿ Polk (1867–1924) designed No. 1019 for the artist Doris Williams (notice the high, half-moon window in her north-facing studio). As part of his fee, he was given the adjoining lot. Here he built No. 1013 for himself in 1892. The house drops down through six levels and is now divided into three apartments.

◢ In 1915 Laura Ingalls Wilder, who wrote the Little House series (the best known volume of which is *Little House on the Prairie*), came to San Francisco to see the Panama-Pacific International Exposition. She stayed with her daughter, Rose, a feature writer for the *San Francisco Bulletin,* who lived at No. 1019. Laura wrote letters home to her husband, Almanzo, in Missouri about the fair, the city, the people, and life on Russian Hill. These letters have been collected in a small paperback titled *West from Home.*

Horatio Gates Livermore walked from St. Joseph, Missouri, to San Francisco in 1850.

◢ The open space at the top of the hill was the 50-vara lot (a California *vara* roughly equals 33 inches) that Horatio Livermore bought in 1889. In 1914, after the residents had subscribed $25,000 for the balustrades and ramps that Polk designed on the Jones side, the top of the summit became the carriage turnaround.

◢ The story of the Polk-designed Vallejo Stairway, which you descend, is one of concerted effort by neighbors over a period of many years to beautify and maintain the surrounding gardens. To continue within the historic context of the neighborhood, they replaced 14 replicas of early lamps (now with halogen bulbs) and installed benches for resting and viewing. This project was the inspiration for the Los Angeles Los Feliz neighborhood's major stairway and ceramic mural wall renovation project in 2000.

◢ Enter the Ina Coolbrith Park (dedicated in 1911), across the street from No. 1715 Taylor, to descend to Mason. Ina Coolbrith (1841–1928), whose uncle Joseph Smith founded the Mormon Church, came to San Francisco from Illinois at the age of 10 in the first covered-wagon train that crossed the Sierra Nevada via Beckwourth Pass. She taught school and later became a librarian at the Bohemian Club and the Oakland Public Library. Although she was honored as poet laureate of California in 1915, her main contribution to the San Francisco literary world was as a catalyst to aspiring writers. Joaquin Miller, George Sterling, Bret Harte, Gelett Burgess, and others met regularly at her home (1067 Broadway) for readings.

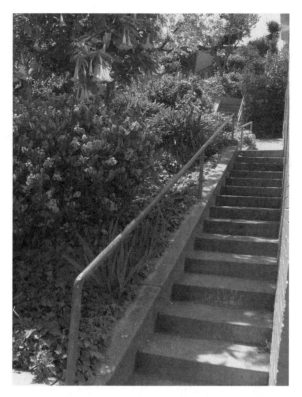

Vallejo Stairway   *Adah Bakalinsky*

◢ Many elderly Chinese come to the park daily to practice Tai Chi. Their mental concentration and slow body movements echo the harmony conveyed by the surrounding canopy of Monterey pines.

◢ At Mason you're on the edge of Chinatown and Russian Hill. Turn right for one block, then right again on Broadway. Notice how the land dips and rises, extending to the highest point south, Nob Hill (see Walk 3).

◢ You are now above the Broadway Tunnel, which extends under Russian Hill from Mason to Larkin. Although the tunnel was proposed in 1874 to facilitate the flow of traffic, it opened for vehicular traffic in 1952—78 years later!

◢ Walk across Broadway to No. 1483 Mason to see the 69-unit Lady Shaw Senior Center, completed in late 1990. The center was financed by her husband, Sir Run Run Shaw, and his brother, Run Me Shaw, through their Shaw Foundation, which supports education, welfare, medicine, and the arts, with a particular emphasis on aiding the elderly, and is one of the largest foundations in the world. Building above the tunnel was controversial, but the critical need for housing in Chinatown, the fine design by architect Gordon Chong & Associates, and the infusion of private, city, and federal funding were decisive factors in favor of construction.

◢ Return to Broadway and turn left. At No. 906, you will see the twin-towered former Spanish National Church, Nuestra Señora de Guadalupe. The 1912 structure is built on the site of the original 1875 wood church.

◢ At the northwest corner of Broadway and Taylor, there is a high retaining wall with decorative edging along the top. Grading of the slopes in the 1860s and 1870s created vertical bluffs. When the streets were lowered, retaining walls and stairways became necessary to protect the houses perched on the top. Walk up the sidewalk stairway on the south side of Broadway for a better view of No. 1020, located up high and toward the back of the property. Albert Farr designed this two-story, brown-shingle, Craftsman-style house in 1909.

◢ Ascend the Florence Stairway next to No. 1032 Broadway. The concrete wall is topped with spindle decoration and a brass plaque (sometimes under cascading vines) that states, "Atkinson-Nichols Landmark Building—1858." There's something strange about this stairway: As you approach each landing, the landscape also seems to rise. Nos. 35, 37, and 39 Florence are Pueblo Revival–style with stucco exteriors and deep-set window apertures to deflect the sun. Robert A. Stern has redesigned No. 40, the original Livermore house on Florence.

◢ When you reach Vallejo (Gelett Burgess lived at No. 1071 for three years), cross the street into Russian Hill Place. Nos. 1, 3, 5, and 7 Russian Hill Place, designed by Willis Polk, were built for Norman Livermore in 1913. It's hard to believe that Russian Hill possesses such a concentration of bewitching little streets in such a small area!

◢ Return to Vallejo, and turn right to walk down the ramp to Jones; turn right to Green, and make a left turn. Walk on the south side, the odd-numbered side. The 1000 block of Green was spared from the earthquake and fire of 1906, so it's architecturally notable. No. 1039–43 is an Italianate of the 1880s and was moved here after 1906. No. 1040 was once the home of the Folger family, whose fortune was made from importing, roasting, and packaging coffee. No. 1055 dates from 1866 and was later remodeled by Julia Morgan. The beautiful carriage house at the rear is now used as living quarters.

◢ You can also see the 1858 octagonal house, the oldest in the city, at No. 1067. A cupola was added in the 1880s. Octagon houses were in vogue for a while because they were purported to be beneficial to your health and sexual vigor. (If you wish to tour the interior of an octagonal house, check the hours of the Colonial Dames Octagon at No. 2645 Gough or call 415-441-7512.) Engine Company No. 31 formerly occupied the 1907 Tudor Revival–style firehouse across the street, which is now a National Trust property.

◢ When you reach Hyde, turn right and then left on Union, the center of the neighborhood shopping area. Across the street, No. 1200 Hyde was Home Drug, where various members of the same family operated the store from 1911 to 1994. The Searchlight Market has been here for a century with various owners. The original Swensen's Ice Cream, here since 1948, still makes the sweet treat on the premises. These shopkeepers provide continuity and stability that contribute to the intangible that is Russian Hill.

◢ Continue west on Union to Polk, and turn right to Greenwich to your beginning.

Further Rambling

If you wish to link with Russian Hill North (Walk 5), begin at Polk and Lombard, and follow the directions in Walk 5.

San Francisco Architectural Signatures

Russian Hill North

From the vantage point of Pacific Heights, Russian Hill appears to be shaped like a square-toed shoe. Coincidentally, many sections of Russian Hill are accessible only to walkers. The redwood-shingled, Craftsman-style homes, designed by Northern California architects Julia Morgan, Willis Polk, and Bernard Maybeck in the early 1900s, blend well into this terrain. Irregularly shaped, deep lots abound; some houses (the kind Adah calls "tuck-ins") are almost invisible from the street. These tuck-ins are as much a part of the city's architectural signature as the loftier towers you see on this walk.

Most hills in San Francisco have either been dug into for rock or bored into for transportation. Abner Doble in 1863 was granted rights to build the Broadway Tunnel through Russian Hill, but he never exercised those rights. In 1952, nearly 80 years later, for about $6 million, the yellow, tiled, two-lane tunnel was completed. Walk through it on the pedestrian paths on either side of the lanes, which were made safer when they were elevated above the car lanes and given sturdy handrails. Enter at either Mason or Larkin at Broadway.

Before or after your walk, hop on a cable car line and take a ride on the running boards (but do hold on). The Powell-Hyde and Powell-Mason cable car lines both run through this walk.

WALK FACTS

The 1931 mural at the San Francisco Art Institute, by Diego Rivera, entitled *The Making of a Fresco Showing the Building of a City,* is worth the visit for the viewing. A fresco within a fresco that takes up the entire end wall of the institute's gallery, it depicts famous engineers, architects, and artists responsible for creating significant artworks in San Francisco.

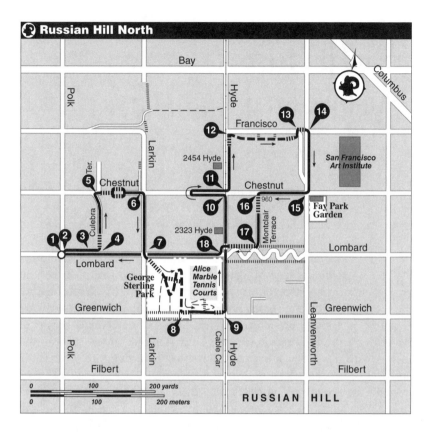

The Norwegian Seaman's Church, at 2454 Hyde near Francisco, opened in 1950 and offers a lovely view of the Bay for fireworks in July. Step in and buy some Norwegian candy (open Tuesday–Sunday, 11 a.m.–5 p.m., closed Mondays).

If you connect Walks 4 and 5, check out the etched tree murals done by Moose Curtis in 2010 near the Broadway Tunnel.

Bus Routes & Parking

PUBLIC TRANSPORTATION: MUNI Bus #19 Polk; #47 and #49 Van Ness. For MUNI bus information, call 311 (outside San Francisco, call 415-701-2311).

PARKING: There is metered street parking available; metered parking is usually for up to an hour, and free street parking is usually allowed for up to two hours. But also look for street-cleaning times posted in the neighborhood to avoid getting ticketed or towed.

QUICK-STEP INSTRUCTIONS

1. Begin at Polk and Lombard, right side of street at No. 1299 Lombard.
2. Cross Lombard to walk up left (north) side of the street.
3. Continue to Culebra Terrace sign at No. 1250.
4. Descend Culebra Terrace Stairway.
5. Right up Chestnut Stairway to Larkin.
6. Right on Larkin. Continue on Larkin to Lombard.
7. Ascend stairway to George Sterling Park. Bear left on path to Greenwich Stairway.
8. Left on stairway to Hyde.
9. Left on Hyde to Lombard. Continue to Chestnut.
10. Detour to 1000 block of Chestnut to view architecture of houses.
11. Return to Hyde and turn left.
12. Right at Francisco. Walk on right upper pedestrian sidewalk toward Leavenworth.
13. Descend stairway. Turn left and descend opposite stairway to Leavenworth.
14. Right on Leavenworth to Chestnut.
15. Right on Chestnut to No. 960.
16. Ascend stairway to Montclair Terrace and continue to Lombard.
17. Right turn on Lombard. Ascend sidewalk stairway to Hyde.
18. Continue on Lombard to Polk to your beginning.

WALK 5 DESCRIPTION

◢ We begin at the corner of Polk and No. 1299 Lombard, built in 1928. The eye-catching ceramic-tiled step risers, decorative metal on the doors, and bas-relief on the pillars provide a dramatic beginning to our exploration of the neighborhood. The 1200 block of Lombard beautifully illustrates the congeniality between the interspersed Italianates and Craftsman-style homes, and between the homes and their hillside location. In this block are several "invisibles," homes that are landlocked and better seen from across the street.

◢ Cross Lombard to view No. 1275, a large shingled Italianate, and Nos. 1267–1263, redwood-shingled refurbished Victorians of 1877. Nos. 1249–1251, a San Francisco Stick Italianate, is a beautiful flat-front tuck-in with a staircase. Built on a hill, it is doubly imposing with its tall false front. No. 1257 is truly a tuck-in and almost hidden. These were all built in 1877 and 1878.

In 1821 at the age of 60, Adam Link walked from his home in Pennsylvania to Ohio (141 miles in three days).

◢ Opposite No. 1251 Lombard, descend the Culebra Terrace Stairway. The hard-to-see sign is on the side of No. 1250. This is a stairway with 29 steps, three landings, and a coda of two steps.

◢ Culebra Terrace is a charming alley of flats and single dwellings enhanced by trees, shrubbery, and flowers. What gives the alley cohesiveness is the combination and proximity of house colors that interact with one another from shades of terra-cotta to yellow. Built in 1911, No. 23 is one of the oldest in the alley. No. 35 has the simplicity of a child's drawing of a house and window. No. 50 has a curved second story of five windows. No. 60 has a terrazzo stairway and decorative small tiles that you can see from the glass door. But as you look at the exterior, you may see a sculpted dragonfly high in the middle of the wall. The smaller one is on the lower right-hand side of the wall. The creator of the sculpture is Arthur McLaughlin. You emerge from Culebra onto the Chestnut cul-de-sac.

◢ Across the street is No. 1154 Chestnut, a villa built in 1913 by a Canadian silver mine owner. Two curved stairways, embellished with handsome, wrought iron railings, partially encircle a flowing fountain that predominates the entrance to the front of the house. This abode is purported to be the first residence in San Francisco to use steel-reinforced concrete in its structure. There are four sycamore trees planted in front of the house. This house also has historical significance, as the residence of Edwin and Irma Grabhorn for 50 years, who started Grabhorn Press of San Francisco.

◢ Grabhorn Press was and is still considered one of the finest small letterpresses in the world, as it continues in its present locations on Hays and in the Presidio National Trust. After the death of the Grabhorn brothers, the Grabhorn Institute was organized in 2000, and in 2002, the California Heritage Council recognized the institute for their work in "preservation of the last fully functioning type foundry and integrated letterpress printing facility." The National Trust for Historic Preservation also calls the institute part of "the nation's irreplaceable historical and cultural legacy" under its Save America's Treasures program. The institute preserves typography and bookmaking that cannot be matched anywhere else in the United States; the artistic works of this press are known historically and are still created

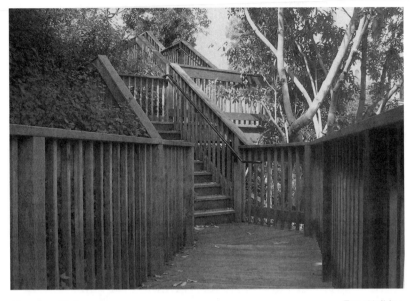

Francisco Stairway *Tony Holiday*

today. Tours are given here on Thursdays at 3 p.m. (the fee is $10). Contact them for reservations at 415-668-2548.

◢ As we turn to ascend the stairway, we see on our right a building, No. 1141, designed with a four-story series of angled sections built to maximize sun and views for the residents.

◢ Walk up the wide Chestnut Stairway shadowed by Canary Island pines and Italian stone pines. Neighbors maintain the landscaping around you. Now, in 48 steps, your amblings bring you to a landing where a U-shaped, double stairway begins. From the landing, you can see one of two dominant landmarks in this section of the city—the unmistakable dome of the Palace of Fine Arts (see Walk 8).

◢ Walk up the left stairway to Larkin. Looking back down the Chestnut corridor, you can see the Presidio ahead of you, as you gaze into the northwest corner of San Francisco, the last piece of mixed open space and commercial and nonprofit real estate people cross through before they leave northward on the Golden Gate Bridge.

◢ Turn right on Larkin. An apartment house on the corner has a brass plaque: "2677 Larkin at Chestnut." (Unfortunately, the architect's name and the date are not cited.)

▄ Continue one block to Lombard. At the corner, walk up the stairway into George Sterling Park, named for a poet who lived in Russian Hill during the 1920s. He is remembered for his description of San Francisco as the "cool gray city of love." Two plaques about him are located at the bottom of the stairway. The low-lying trunks of myrtle trees and the nodules of exposed roots along the path give you a feeling of entering ancient woods. A bench has been thoughtfully placed to permit a meditative view northwest to the Marin hills.

▄ Bear left up the stairs past the bench (to the sound above of tennis balls against racquets). The next landing is Phoebe's Terrace (named for a neighborhood benefactor). Pass the mosaic-tile wall, and then walk right on the sidewalk. Watch for posted signs: "Be Coyote Aware." White crown sparrows seem to have the air rights around here—perfect acoustics for their beautiful song and perfect sighting for their gliding and dipping flights. Tennis and basketball players gradually come into view on the left. A plaque for Phoebe Terrace is on the concrete post as you approach the Greenwich Stairway.

▄ Turn left to ascend the stairway and explore the stone terraced ramps and landscaping leading to the tennis courts. The San Francisco Public Utilities Commission restored the park in 2005. The

Lombard Street   *Tony Holiday*

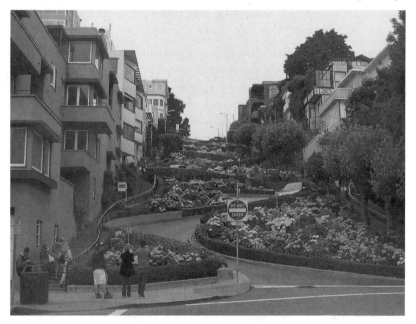

Alice Marble Tennis Courts, also part of the 2.6-acre park, are on San Francisco Public Utilities Commission land, with the Lombard Reservoir beneath (built in 1860) supplying six to eight surrounding blocks. Born in the small California town of Dutch Flat, Alice Marble (1913–1990) spent some of her adolescent years in San Francisco. She joined the Golden Gate Park Tennis Club, a training ground for many outstanding players and, during 1936–1940, was a four-time winner of the National Women's Singles Tennis championship. A plaque tells of the rededication of the reservoir to her in 2005.

⊿ Descend 26 steps to Hyde, turn left to face Alcatraz (another San Francisco signature), and continue to Lombard. No. 2222 is an eight-story steel-framed, reinforced-concrete cooperative (1920), one of five constructed by T. Paterson Ross in this Russian Hill neighborhood. His buildings are rich in interior detail and utilize the latest technology of their era of construction. Ross designed about 200 buildings during a 32-year period. When he sustained brain injuries from falling bricks in an open freight elevator while inspecting the Union League Club, his professional career ended. He was 49 then, but lived to be 84.

⊿ The intersection of Hyde and Lombard is a splendid place to stop and see the Hyde Street Cable Car lurching along with its standing-room-only crowd of passengers. Accorded the conductor's full approval, they alight en masse with their cameras pointed toward Alcatraz, Coit Tower, the Bay Bridge, or Treasure Island. At the clang of the cable car bell, they rush aboard once more to coast down to the next landing on their way to Aquatic Park. No. 2323 Hyde, across the street, is a Willis Polk house designed for Robert Louis Stevenson's widow, Fanny, who lived there from 1899 to 1908. (Lombard and Hyde was purported to be Stevenson's favorite San Francisco corner.) The structure is now an apartment house.

⊿ Continue walking north on Hyde to Chestnut. An inappropriately placed high-rise on the corner still suffers that friendless look. Previously this was the site (No. 998 Chestnut) of the landmark 12-room house built in 1852 by William Clark, who built the first wharf near the foot of Broadway (Walk 1).

⊿ Detour left on Chestnut to experience the ambiance of the 1000 block. Between Nos. 1000 and 1080 is a delightful series of three-story, mansard-roofed homes painted in pastel colors. The south side of the street features the back entrance of the award-winning Lombardia complex, 10 large town houses and 32 condos designed by well-known architects Hood and Miller (on a lot that was vacant for

28 years). By thoughtful use of scale, space, light, and plant materials, they created an inviting Mediterranean setting. No. 1089 Chestnut, completed in 1990, has 17-foot ceilings in the living room and 5,600 square feet of space.

▪ Return to Hyde, turn left (north), and walk on the right side of the street past the Norwegian Seaman's Church at No. 2454 Hyde. From the left side of Hyde, you can see the roof of another reservoir. Straight ahead (north) is the Hyde St. Pier with its famous collection of historic ships. At Francisco turn right and walk on the upper pedestrian sidewalk toward Leavenworth.

▪ The Francisco cul-de-sac is a beauty, a true favorite. The large homes here, designed in a variety of architectural styles, are set on several levels of land that command enviable views from either side of the street.

▪ The frame two-story at No. 825 is originally dated 1849 but has undergone many renovations. It was constructed of timber salvaged from ships abandoned in the Bay during the Gold Rush. No. 828 Francisco, at the end of the cul-de-sac, has a bay of leaded windows with octagonal inserts, a modified mansard roof, and beautiful copper chimney stacks, which have acquired a greenish cast over the years. A fence espaliered that hosts flat, fragrant jasmine follows the slope of the hill.

▪ From the parapet next to No. 800 Francisco, you can gaze at the variety of geometric shapes and signatures that are part of a San Franciscan's daily eyeful: the abundant, sword-shaped leaves of a palm tree at the lower corner of the street, the square Romanesque tower of the San Francisco Art Institute, the rectangular towers of the Bay Bridge, the conical towers of Saints Peter and Paul Church in North Beach, the cylindrical Coit Tower, and the pyramidal Transamerica building.

▪ Descend the short stairway to the street. Cross to the opposite side of Francisco, and descend the stairway to Leavenworth. Walk across Leavenworth, and turn right to Chestnut. At the corner of Leavenworth, detour a few steps to Fay Park Garden at No. 2366 Leavenworth. San Francisco was the recent recipient of this property owned by the Fay family. It is distinguished by a Thomas Church garden that was designed for the family in 1957 and includes trees, flowers, and gazebos. The garden is now open to the public; however, the mansion is not, at this time.

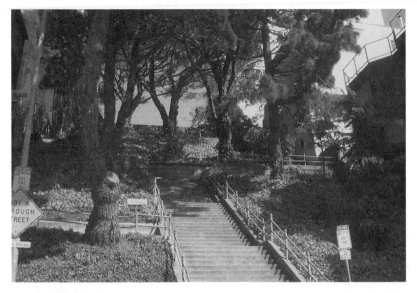

Chestnut Stairway   *Tony Holiday*

⊿ Turn right on Chestnut. No. 930 has a flat roof, while No. 944, built in 1864, has columns and a balcony. Across the street from No. 960, ascend 28 steps to Montclair Terrace, a hidden court of homes and gardens. No. 66, designed in 1956 by one of Adah's favorite architects, Henry Hill, has simplicity and flourish. Next to No. 4 you're at Lombard, where drivers enjoy the unusual ride down the most photographed, photogenic, hairpin-turn street in the country: eight turns within an 800-foot-long section and a grade of 18.18%. City Engineer Preston Wallace King designed it in 1922, from a 26% grade, cobblestoned Lombard.

⊿ Turn right on Lombard to walk up a straight, comfortable stairway. At the top, continue west on Lombard to Polk to your beginning.

North Waterfront: A Segmented Metamorphosis o'er Land & Sea

Fort Mason

The north waterfront neighborhood hugging Fort Mason and the Marina offers amazing views and great opportunities for enjoying the parks with many other families and tourists around you. Even cable cars aren't too far away. But here, you can relive what the waterfront was used for: a dump, a rifle range, and finally, a great environmental research center for the San Francisco community. Museums, artists' studios, and, as always, great food all bring their own unique charms to this edge of the salty Bay and its briny lapping waters.

On this walk you explore some of the extensive municipal and federal recreational areas of San Francisco along its northern waterfront. Walking west from Marina Green through Presidio lands or east from the Marina Green to the Hyde St. Pier, you can appreciate how this land became a focus for federal military installations and then slowly evolved, under the aegis of the Department of the Interior, into land for a national park. The area you traverse is part of the Golden Gate National Recreation Area (GGNRA), the most popular urban park in the United States. More apparent here than in other neighborhoods is how the continuum of history blends into an evolving contemporary scene. Naturally, the atmosphere is highly energized.

WALK FACTS

This walk offers excellent wide-open views of the Bay, Angel and Alcatraz Islands, and the North and East Bays beyond. It afforded some of the most dramatic views for watching the 2013 America's Cup yacht races involving teams from New Zealand, Italy, and Norway, as well as the Oracle Team representing America.

The Aquatic Bathhouse and Maritime Museum was originally built as the area's main building and included an emergency hospital, banquet rooms, sunrooms, and a lounge.

Bus Routes & Parking

PUBLIC TRANSPORTATION: MUNI Bus #28 19th Ave. For MUNI bus information, call 311 (outside San Francisco, call 415-701-2311).

PARKING: Parking is available at Gashouse Cove or Marina Green, as well as inside the gate at Fort Mason for a fee.

WALK 6 DESCRIPTION

◢ Begin on the Gashouse Cove Marina path, and enter Fort Mason by the side of Building A. (Pick up a calendar of events at the Fort Mason Foundation office, or call 415-441-3400.) For many years this was the point of embarkation for men and supplies. The Army used the buildings alongside the piers through demobilization after World War II and the Korean War. They are now used for recreational and cultural activities. Lower Fort Mason, which is managed and administered by the nonprofit Fort Mason Foundation, is the headquarters for more than 50 nonprofit community and cultural organizations, including theaters, museums, music schools, dance studios, computer groups, the Children's Art Center, and Lawyers for the Arts. The Greens Restaurant in Building A, an outstanding vegetarian restaurant, has been here since 1979. Its seating offers a view of the Bay and the Golden Gate Bridge.

◢ Walk toward the water and then to your right. You pass Buildings A, B, C, D, and E; Pier 1; Pier 2, the Herbst Pavilion, and the Cowell Theater; Pier 3; and the Festival Pavilion. The J. Porter Shaw Maritime Library in Building E is open to the general public Monday through Friday by appointment; call 415-561-7030. As you walk along the wall, note the stern of the *Galilee*, a Tahitian trading vessel, built in 1891 and in use until 1920. The Oceanic Society has offices nearby. San Francisco City College and the Long Now Foundation have also rented space in Fort Mason.

◢ Opposite Building E is a stairway. You may see hummingbirds dipping and revolving around one another in their courtship ritual as you walk up it. A Monterey cypress is on the left.

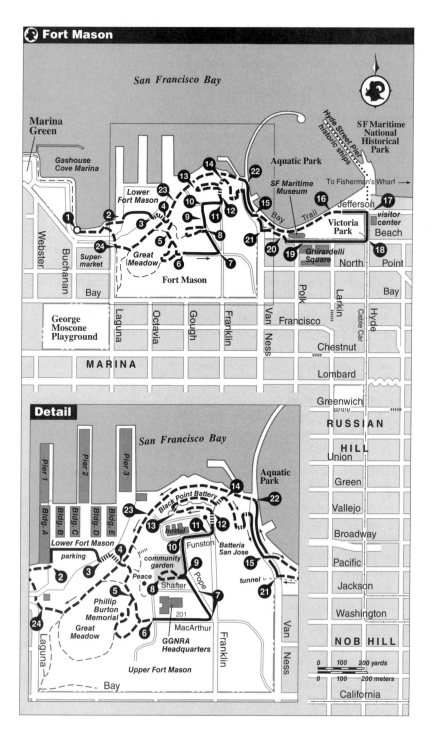

QUICK-STEP INSTRUCTIONS

1. Begin at Gashouse Cove.
2. Walk on sidewalk along waterfront to the side of Building A in lower Fort Mason.
3. Ascend the stairway opposite Building E.
4. Walk on any of the paths around or through the Great Meadow.
5. Pass Bufano *Madonna* sculpture. Pass *Phillip Burton Memorial.*
6. Left on MacArthur to park headquarters (Building No. 201).
7. Continue on to Pope past Shafter, and then go left at Building 204.
8. Walk around the Community Garden and out on Pope.
9. Left on Pope.
10. Right on Funston.
11. Left on Franklin.
12. Walk to the end of Franklin and descend stairway.
13. Left and walk around Black Point Battery. Ascend wood stairway to upper level.
14. Right on footpath at top of wall. Descend stairways and walkways to Van Ness. Turn right.
15. Cross Van Ness. Turn right and then left on promenade.
16. Continue on promenade to Jefferson and Hyde.
17. Right on Hyde to Beach.
18. Right on Beach to Polk.
19. Continue across Polk and past the Maritime Museum. Veer left past low white wall and benches.
20. Descend stairway. Turn left and walk railroad-track path to Van Ness.
21. Right on Van Ness to the pier.
22. At pier, turn left to ascend paved path.
23. Follow path through Great Meadow to Laguna.
24. At bottom of hill, across from Safeway, you are at your beginning.

The next level at Fort Mason features former military housing, the International Hostel, and the GGNRA headquarters—a resource for information about the entire national park system, as well as community conservation issues. (For more information, call 415-561-4700.) The National Park Service continually monitors problem areas. They plant soil-huggers like sand verbena, ice plant, and dune daisy to restrain the constantly shifting, sandy soil. They build stairways to prevent erosion, preserve the fragile topsoil, and keep people on the trails.

◢ Turn around to see Marina Blvd., the Golden Gate Bridge, and the Marin Headlands. Take the path to the left, walking counterclockwise toward the Great Meadow. You are retracing the long-forgotten footsteps of hundreds of men, women, and children who lived here in tents after losing their homes in the 1906 earthquake. Refugee Camp No. 5 extended west beyond the meadow to the site of the present Safeway store. Fort Mason was an important site during and after the 1906 earthquake. The Navy fireboat anchored here was used to pump water from the Bay to the fire engines along Van Ness. Fort Mason was the headquarters for General Frederick Funston, who had to put San Francisco under martial law to prevent looting. Subsequently, under General Adolphus Washington Greely, it became the relief-supply distribution center. When Mayor Eugene Schmitz moved his office here, Fort Mason became the center for coordinating civil and military authority.

◢ Following the paved footpath to the right, you reach the Beniamino Bufano sculpture of cast stone and mosaic dedicated to and named *Madonna*. A favorite San Francisco personality, Bufano (1898–1970) was supported by various benefactors, such as the owner of the Powell restaurant (now defunct) for which he designed and executed a mosaic mural in return for a lifetime of meals.

◢ Walk along the path to the *Phillip Burton Memorial*, designed by landscape architect Tito Patri; the project sculptor was Wendy Ross. The 10-foot sculpture of Burton represents him in his everyday look— wearing rumpled trousers, making an emphatic gesture, his jacket pocket holding a scribbled note for later. In 1983, Congress dedicated the GGNRA to Congressman Burton, who was responsible for the federal legislation that made the park a reality. The sculpture was unveiled in the spring of 1991. (If you look to the right, you can see the Palace of Fine Arts dome and the Golden Gate Bridge.)

◢ Continue east on the path to the park headquarters, Building No. 201, on MacArthur. It was built in 1901 as a military hospital. After the 1906 earthquake, it was used as an emergency center and a lying-in hospital. According to legend, eight babies were born at Fort Mason the night after the quake.

◢ In the years following 1906, Building No. 201 was used as administrative headquarters for Fort Mason. During World War II Ronald Reagan (president of the United States, 1981–89) served here as second lieutenant in charge of tracking down missing shipments. Fort Mason was declared a National Historic Landmark in 1985.

⊿ Make a sharp left turn on Pope to pass around the headquarters. To your right, near the corner of Franklin, are the Mission Revival–style Chapel (1942) and the starting place of the Conversation-Pace Game field, sponsored by the San Francisco Senior Center. Various exercises here are paced slowly enough to allow for conversation.

⊿ Continue on Pope past Shafter. At Building 204 turn left on the sidewalk into the gated Community Garden to explore greenhouses, lattice works, and terraces and to view the enormous variety of plants, vegetables, and flowers in cultivation. Several of the gardeners specialize in rare varieties of flowers. The Fort Mason garden is very popular and, even though space is available to anyone who applies, the average wait time is five years. Return to Pope, and go left.

⊿ The San Francisco International Hostel at the end of Pope, Building 240, formerly a Civil War barracks built in 1863, is a friendly, clean, and inviting place. You may see some of the guests out about on the grass, or reading. The hostel can accommodate 151 guests and has nine private rooms; there is 24-hour access and no curfew.

⊿ From the hostel turn right on Funston, passing the sign for Building 240. Continue to Franklin, and walk across to the area interpretive sign. This part of Fort Mason contains military residences dating from the 1850s. The officers' housing on the east side of Pope originated as squatters' homes, put up in the same period by prominent San Franciscans who understood the value of the real estate. Shortly afterward the Army took possession of the homes and began building fortifications in anticipation of a Confederate attack.

⊿ Strong pro- and anti-slavery feelings in California culminated in the famous Terry–Broderick duel in 1859. Senator David Broderick, shot by the hot-tempered, pro-slavery Judge David Terry near Lake Merced, died here at Fort Mason in the home of a friend. The Haskell House interpretive sign is to the right.

⊿ Continue left on Franklin along the concrete walkway. You pass the Palmer House erected in 1855. Then you reach an open green space on the left, where John Fremont's home was from 1859 to 1861. The upper area was also the site of the Batteria San Jose, a Spanish seacoast defense battery located here in 1797. It was built to protect the Yerba Buena anchorage, later known as Black Point Cove (1820s) and now known as Aquatic Park. Black Point Cove was once part of the San Jose Point Military Reservation, which became Fort Mason in 1882.

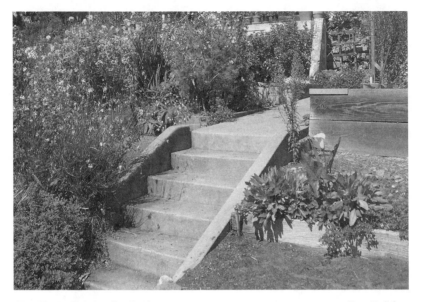

Fort Mason Community Garden   *Tony Holiday*

⊿ This particular area was important to the Spanish, Mexicans, and Americans because its strategic location made it ideal for defense. Theoretically, the Bay was well defended against hostile fleets. At one time or another, there were Spanish or American coastal batteries on the Marin Headlands, Alcatraz, Angel Island, Fort Point, and here at Fort Mason. The best preserved of these antiquated defenses is Fort Point, the Civil War fort under the arch of the Golden Gate Bridge.

⊿ Walk to the end of Franklin, and descend the stairway to the picnic area and Black Point Battery. You are standing on what is known as Black Point Lookout, so-called because of the dark vegetation provided by the laurel trees. The picnic area was constructed on this battery platform, which dates to the Civil War. There are four tables and benches where you can sit to enjoy food and the sublime view, which, when Adah last visited, featured a procession of boats with multicolored sails of pink, green, and blue, backlit against the clearly delineated hills of Marin and the East Bay. My last visit was crowded with spectators for the America's Cup race, but weekdays are often freer, with many walkers, joggers, and strollers bustling nearby. To use the tables, make a reservation by calling 415-561-4300.

⊿ Walk across the area of the battery emplacements in the wall on your left. At the western end is a 10-ton cannon. The sign reads

"1863 Battery." Another emplacement sign reads "1898 Battery," both part of Black Point Battery. This site was excavated from 1981 to 1983. The land is stabilized with no further excavations planned. To your left is a native plant habitat. Ascend the railroad-tie steps to the wall of the battery. Turn right and walk back to the picnic area.

⚓ Turn left to descend the stairway. As you turn right to walk the long, paved walkway, these are some of the sights that come into view: the East Bay; both spans of the Bay Bridge connected by Yerba Buena Island; Treasure Island, the long strip of land left of Yerba Buena; Fisherman's Wharf; the long pedestrian pier at the end of Van Ness; the Cannery; and Hyde Street Pier with historic ships. Continue on the walkway, where concrete and stone benches have conveniently been placed. When you pass a gate that leads to a private residence, bear left down the stairways, and take the walkway to Van Ness.

⚓ Cross the extension of Van Ness to get to the edge of the water in Aquatic Park. There are public restrooms in the white structure, decorated with incised, wavy lines near the roof to simulate ocean waves, an example of the Streamline Moderne–style of the 1930s. (The twin of this structure is located at the end of Jefferson.) Take the walkway just before the public restrooms. Walk on the promenade along the water, and ascend the amphitheater steps to watch birds and swimmers. The inviting sandy beach we enjoy today was originally a dismal beach of gravel and seaweed. It was renovated with tons of sand taken from Union Square when an underground garage was built there in the 1930s.

Samuel Taylor Coleridge walked 10 miles daily and worked out the setting of The Rime of the Ancient Mariner *on a walking tour with William Wordsworth.*

⚓ The ship-shaped building to the right, originally Aquatic Park Bathhouse, is a Works Progress Administration project completed in 1939, which is now the Maritime Museum, founded by Karl Kortum in 1950. The street-level floor has restored murals, tile work, and terrazzo floors; it is open and available for viewing. The Aquatic Park Senior Center, active since 1947, also uses part of the building. The first and second floors of the museum are open from 9:30 a.m. to 5 p.m. daily. The third floor is also now open for exhibits, which change from time to time.

⚓ Walk east on Jefferson, passing the Dolphin Swimming and Boating Club established in 1877. Members still swim in the Bay. Next to it is the South End Rowing Club.

⬛ Historic ships are docked at the Hyde St. Pier, and you can take an imaginary trip: on the *Eureka* ferry, you'd board as a passenger; on the *Thayer,* as a sailor manning this schooner, which carried lumber, salmon, and codfish; or if you're the ruddier sort of matey, perhaps the *Balclutha,* a square-rigger known to cut fast on the ocean in calm or storm. A nominal fee to board the ships helps defray the expense of preserving them. The bookstore has an excellent collection pertaining to the sea and related subjects.

⬛ At the corner of Hyde and Jefferson, cross the street to the San Francisco Maritime National Historical Park Visitor Center, which has exhibits of local maritime history. It opens daily at 9:30 a.m. and is staffed by park rangers. You may enjoy a visit next door at the cannery for shopping and browsing.

⬛ Walk up Hyde along the side of Victoria Park (designed by Thomas Church in 1960), which is festive with a gazebo and flowers, and the cable car turntable. Jovial crowds of tourists and residents are often waiting to board.

⬛ Turn right on Beach. Musicians and performers are interspersed among the outdoor stall displays of jewelry, T-shirts, leather belts, pen-and-ink drawings of San Francisco scenes, and stained-glass mobiles and window insets.

⬛ Continue to Larkin. Ghirardelli Square, at the corner, is a pioneer example of adaptive use. In this case, the former chocolate factory, which was built in 1893, was converted in 1967 into a well-designed complex of residences, fine-quality specialty shops, and restaurants.

⬛ Continue on Beach, and cross Polk. Walk past the Maritime Museum and the low wall and benches. Descend the stairway to the promenade. Turn left on the railroad-track path back to Van Ness. Across the street is the tunnel, bored into the rocks under Fort Mason, through which the Belt Line Railroad tracks ran. The Belt Line, opened in 1896, covered the city front from Islais Creek to the Presidio. Its original purpose was to move boxcars and flatcars directly alongside cargo vessels. In the late 1920s, it transported men and military supplies to the Presidio; in the late 1950s, the military filled in the tracks.

⬛ Turn right on Van Ness, and walk along the curved concrete wall of Aquatic Park to the pier. Pumping Station No. 2, built to supply water in case of earthquake and fire, is on the left side of the street. Opposite, you can see the small, fenced wood section of what was formerly the Alcatraz Pier. Here, convicts boarded a boat for the island prison.

⊿ Turn left and walk up the paved path to the Great Meadow. Along the way, you will see Alcatraz, Angel Island, the Golden Gate Bridge, and even Marin (if it isn't foggy). If you look down the path behind you, you will see the original rocky shoreline.

⊿ Continue through the meadow to Laguna and Gashouse Cove to your beginning.

Further Rambling

From the Marina Green at Scott and Marina, follow the path to the water, and turn left onto the Coastal Trail to reach the lovingly restored Crissy Field. This 20-acre tidal marsh, shoreline promenade, and restored dunes and beach circle the community environmental center built here in 2001. (Prior to 1915, the US Army used Crissy Field as a dump; in the 1920s, the space was used for an airfield and a rifle range.) You can continue on this trail up to Fort Point, built in 1861 for defense against the South during the Civil War. Its walls are 7 feet thick and 45 feet high, and it survived the 1906 earthquake. Go have a look.

Retrace your steps to the Crissy Field Trail, then turn left or east toward the San Francisco Yacht Club to reach the Wave Organ at the jetty's end. Peter Richards designed it, and master stonemason and sculptor George Gonzalez built it. When the Exploratorium was still at the Palace of Fine Arts, the shoreline and Crissy Field became part of the activities organized around learning early on. Here you can sit down, enjoy the view of the skyline, and listen to the water music below. This sound garden, built from recycled marble and granite from the dismantled Lone Mountain Cemetery, opened in 1986. Since then, silt has lessened the pipe's cacophony somewhat, but this nearby diversion, the views, and the sounds make for a splendid coda to the walk.

Or if you want to go the other way, follow the promenade along the water, in the direction of Fillmore (west) to Marina Green. There you may see people flying kites, and along the waterfront, you may see coots, western grebes, and mallards. Mallow, oxalis, and tower of jewels bloom beside the walkway, inviting you to take a stroll.

Walks 8 and 29 are nearby too, if you follow the shoreline east and then south. Walk 2 is also just a few blocks to the east, at Bay and Mason. Go ahead; take another stroll.

Walk Forward, But Always Look Back

Pacific Heights

After the first cable car went over Nob Hill in 1878, Pacific Heights, the ridge across the Polk–Van Ness Valley, began to be developed. Then as now, the views of the Bay were extraordinary. Although a precipitous 370 feet above sea level, the heights had many wide, flat lots for the large homes only the wealthy could afford.

WALK FACTS

In July, Pacific Heights participates in the largest outdoor free jazz concert in North America, the Fillmore Jazz Festival. The festival runs for two days, rain or shine, and brings together the Pacific Heights, Japantown, and Western Addition neighborhoods for cool tunes.

Bus Routes & Parking

PUBLIC TRANSPORTATION: MUNI Bus #3 Jackson and #45 Union. For MUNI bus information, call 311 (outside San Francisco, call 415-701-2311).

PARKING: There is metered street parking available; metered parking is usually available for up to an hour, and free street parking is usually allowed for up to two hours. But also look for street-cleaning times posted in the neighborhood to avoid getting ticketed or towed.

WALK 7 DESCRIPTION

◢ Begin at Broadway and Baker. Bliss and Faville, famous for their designs of classical government buildings, built No. 2898 Broadway, on the northeast corner, in 1889. (A few blocks away on Broadway, toward the end of this walk, you will see another Bliss and Faville structure to compare.)

◢ Descend the two-block-long Baker Stairway. Monterey pines and cypresses in the center area and dense shrubs on both sides confine the stairway. In addition, the tread-to-riser proportion of the stairs is not felicitous.

◢ Enter Vallejo. The large home on your left at No. 2901 Vallejo, built in 1886, is a combination of Mediterranean and Mission styles. Turn right to look at Nos. 2881 and 2891, which have extremely narrow second-story windows. These homes were originally connected and were modeled after a church.

◢ Continue on Baker to descend the lower section of the stairway on the right, which feels lighter and more cheerful than the upper section. Open space around the comfortable stairs makes this a happy, bouncy descent. No. 2511 is a redwood-shingled box with a twin-gabled roof.

There is no orthodoxy in walking. It is a land of many paths and no paths, where everyone goes his own way and is right.
—George Macaulay Trevelyan

◢ The Palace of Fine Arts is in the center of the view, surrounded by the North Bay and the circle of hills beyond it. Similar particularly appealing houses at Nos. 2872 and 2880 Green are to our left. Go to the end of the Green St. cul-de-sac to look at the variety and the unity of the architecture and the crown jewel at No. 2601 Lyon.

◢ Come back to the corner of Baker, and continue walking along Green to Pierce. No. 2790 is the Russian Consulate. No. 2452 is a tuck-in; No. 2423 was built in 1891 by the architect Ernest Coxhead, who built his own house next door at No. 2421. No. 2411 has a slate roof.

◢ Turn right on Pierce to No. 2727, an original farm mansion built in 1865 by Henry Casebolt. He was a blacksmith, builder, and inventor. He started the Sutter St. Railway (a horse car line) and invented the balloon car, an early form of the streetcar that was rounded and carried its own turntable. Continue to Broadway.

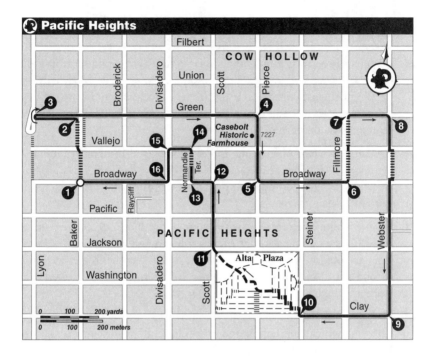

Turn left on Broadway to Fillmore. Descend the Fillmore Stairway on the right side from Broadway to Vallejo. There are spectacular views from the west to the north. Continue descending the stairway from Vallejo to Green. Feel the difference in walking comfort between the stairway on the left, an L-shaped tread, and the one on the right, a sloping tread. No. 2323 Vallejo is the Vedanta Society Temple designed by Henry Gutterson and completed in 1959. The architecture is more subdued than that of the original 1905 temple on Filbert and Webster. Both temples are still in use. The basic philosophic tenet of Vedantism is that all paths to God are equally true. Everything comes from the divine spirit, and the purpose of life is to discover that unfolding spirit within us and everywhere else. Nearby are the monastery and convent, where men and women train to become monastics.

Turn right on Green to Webster. No. 2160 Webster, built in 1867 for Leander Sherman of Sherman Clay music stores, has landmark status. Frequent musical evenings were hosted here. Visiting artists performed, among them Madame Ernestine Schumann-Heink and Ignace Jan Paderewski.

QUICK-STEP INSTRUCTIONS

1. Begin at Baker and Broadway. Descend two-block-long Baker Stairway to Green.
2. Left on Green to view cul-de-sac.
3. Return on Green to Pierce.
4. Right on Pierce to Broadway.
5. Left on Broadway to Fillmore.
6. Left on Fillmore. Descend Fillmore (sidewalk) Stairway on right to Green.
7. Right on Green to Webster.
8. Right on Webster. Ascend Webster (sidewalk) Stairway at Vallejo. Continue to Clay.
9. Right on Clay to Steiner.
10. Ascend the Clay Stairway of Alta Plaza Park. Walk west across the park to Jackson and Scott.
11. Right on Scott to Broadway.
12. Left on Broadway for a half block to Normandie Terrace.
13. Walk to the end of the cul-de-sac. Descend stairway to Vallejo.
14. Left on Vallejo to Divisadero.
15. Left on Divisadero to Broadway.
16. Right on Broadway to Baker to your beginning.

◢ Turn right on Webster to Vallejo, and ascend the stairway to Broadway. At the top look back to see one of San Francisco's many views. Nos. 2120 and 2222 Broadway are two estates that belonged to the Flood family (of Comstock mine fortune) and are now private schools. The former, built in 1898 for James C. Flood, is the Sarah Dix Hamlin School for Girls. The gardens and tennis courts extend the depth of the lot to No. 2129 Vallejo, where an addition to the school was built in 1965; the two buildings are connected by a stairway. No. 2222 Broadway, the Convent of the Sacred Heart High School, was designed in 1912 in memory of James L. Flood's son (also named James) who passed away at age four from a burst appendix (he was the grandson of James C. Flood). This Italian Renaissance–style mansion by Bliss and Faville has an exterior of Tennessee marble; the interior has hand-carved wood paneling of oak, satinwood, and walnut. (Surely the Hebrew tradition of placing honey on the first page of the first book a child reads, to promote sweet associations with learning, applies as well to learning in such beautiful surroundings.)

◢ Though it displays a pineapple finial, a symbol of hospitality, No. 2550 Webster is a heavy looking, uninviting, clinker-brick structure. Willis Polk built it in 1896 for William Bourn, who at various times was head of the Spring Valley Water Company, Pacific Gas & Electric, and the Empire Mining Company in Grass Valley. Polk also designed Filoli, Bourn's garden estate in Woodside, which is now part of the National Trust for Historic Preservation.

◢ The Newcomer High School, formerly at Jackson and Webster has moved to 1350 7th Ave. It provides bilingual classes for almost 90 languages and transitional education for recently arrived immigrant students.

◢ At Nos. 2321–2315 Webster, between Jackson and Washington, are a series of slanted-bay Italianates that date from 1878. Calla lilies and roses growing in the gardens complement the simple character of the houses. In the next block, between Washington and Clay, is a series of attached, slanted-bay Italianates, Nos. 2253–2233. These homes are in the Webster Historic District. Yet another group of Italianates, Nos. 2221–2209, round out the picture of the Victorian community. The California Pacific Medical Center, which presently dominates the

Alta Plaza Park   *Polly Gates*

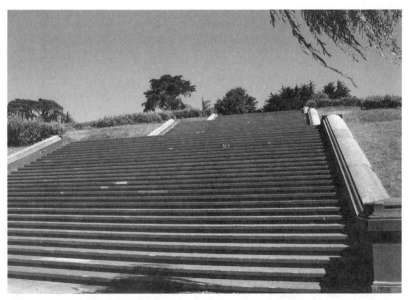

area, has evolved from a merger of the University of the Pacific Medical School and Presbyterian Hospital.

◢ Turn right on Clay. One block ahead to the right is No. 2318 Fillmore, once the site of a stagecoach stop, now the Smith-Kettlewell Eye Research Institute.

◢ At Steiner you walk up the Clay Stairway of Alta Plaza Park, which was purchased in 1877. John McLaren, the superintendent of Golden Gate Park for 60 years, designed the 12 acres of excessively steep Alta Plaza in the only way possible—with slopes and terraces. The stairways are magnificent and the views varied. Looking down from the hill on the row of Italianates on Clay (Nos. 2637–2673), you appreciate the presence and the scale of these post–Civil War structures with their imposing false fronts.

◢ Walk across the park northwest toward Jackson and Scott; continue north on Scott to Broadway. Turn left on Broadway and right into Normandie Terrace, a special enclave of a few custom-designed homes. At the end of the cul-de-sac, descend the stairway. Turn left on Vallejo and left on Divisadero. At Broadway is another view to the east-northeast. Turn right on Broadway, but not before you find the sculpture *Goliath the Robot,* and then continue to Baker to your beginning.

Tripping Lightly

Presidio Wall & Marina Waterfront

On this walk you will trip lightly through adjoining sections of three neighborhoods—Pacific Heights, Letterman Digital Arts Center (George Lucas's film campus), and lower sections of the Marina. You'll experience a contrast in topography, from 379 feet to sea level, and have the comfortable feeling that the neighborhoods fit together after all. Imagine that you're on a vacation stroll or, better yet, an everyday stroll that is alive with beautiful sights for the eyes.

The Presidio, the Marina harbor, the Palace of Fine Arts with its surrounding lagoon and paths area, and Crissy Field's promenade and beaches are magnets attracting people from everywhere to come out and enjoy a day in the city. This area is part of the landfill site of the spectacular Panama-Pacific International Exposition of 1915, celebrating the rebirth of San Francisco after the 1906 earthquake. This extravagant and most classic of fairs signaled to all the world that San Francisco, like the mythical phoenix, had arisen from the ashes of the 1906 earthquake to become again the cool gray city that everybody loves.

WALK FACTS

Parts of the Presidio Wall, which was originally a wood fence that separated the city from the military post, were gradually replaced by a low stone wall.

Houses in this area were mostly built in the late 19th and early 20th century, but Juana Briones and her husband, Apolinario Miranda, a soldier at the Presidio, were deeded the property under the Lyon Street steps and the Agua de Figueroa spring in 1833, where the Presidio Wall stops. After she and her husband divorced, Juana took her fight to keep this land all the way to the Supreme Court, where she ultimately won in 1861, under what came to be known as the Miranda Grant.

Bus Routes & Parking

PUBLIC TRANSPORTATION: MUNI Bus #28 19th Ave., #43 Masonic, and #30 Stockton. For MUNI bus information, call 311 (outside San Francisco, call 415-701-2311).

PARKING: There is metered street parking available; metered parking is usually available for up to an hour, and free street parking is usually allowed for up to two hours. But also look for street-cleaning times posted in the neighborhood to avoid getting ticketed or towed.

WALK 8 DESCRIPTION

◢ Begin your walk at the intersection of Lyon and Gorgas at the Presidio Wall. Turn left on Gorgas. Walk on the sidewalk between the two concrete columns, approximately 7 feet high. Opposite the four short green posts, turn left, and walk through two handsome stone pillars to enter the unusual public garden designed by Lawrence Halprin Associates. This entrance is Gorgas Gate, unmarked at present.

◢ Ascend the stone stairway on the left, and walk under a series of standing metal arches, embellished with cut-steel maple leaves. One time Adah took this walk, the sun was shining, magnified reflections of the patterns were displayed on the sidewalks, and the abundance of field rocks and boulders and their placement—on low walls, alongside the falls, and around the lagoon—caught her attention. They come from the Redding, California, area. The garden imparts a sense of "There is time. You don't have to rush." Much of it likely comes from the rocks.

◢ Ascend the stone slab stairway to the path. At your own pace and direction, follow the paths and areas leading to a cafe and restaurant open to the public and four sculptures by Lawrence Noble: Eadweard Muybridge, the photographer famous for his experiment proving that all four legs of horses are off the ground at one point when running; Philo Farnsworth, inventor of television; Yoda at Building B; and Willis O'Brien, animator of the original *King Kong* movie and stop-motion genius, in Building B (open on weekdays only).

◢ George Lucas was awarded the privilege of leasing land for his film campus, Letterman Digital Arts Center (LDAC), which is, at this time,

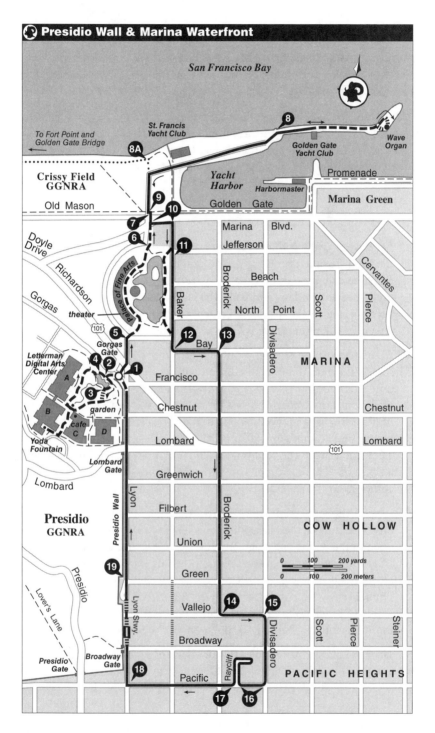

Presidio Wall & Marina Waterfront

San Francisco Bay

To Fort Point and
Golden Gate Bridge

St. Francis
Yacht Club

8

8A

Golden Gate
Yacht Club

Wave
Organ

**Crissy Field
GGNRA**

Old Mason

*Yacht
Harbor*

Promenade

Marina Green

Golden   Gate

Harbormaster

Doyle
Drive

Richardson

9

7

10

6

11

Marina   Blvd.

Jefferson

Gorgas

Palace of Fine Arts

theater

Beach

Baker

Broderick

North   Point

Divisadero

Scott

Cervantes

Pierce

101

5

Gorgas
Gate

12

13

Bay

MARINA

**Letterman
Digital Arts
Center**

4

2

1

A

3

garden

Francisco

Chestnut

Chestnut

B

cafe

C

D

Lombard

Lombard

**Yoda
Fountain**

Lombard
Gate

Greenwich

101

Lombard

Lyon

Filbert

Broderick

Union

COW HOLLOW

**Presidio
GGNRA**

Presidio Wall

Green

0   100   200 yards
0   100   200 meters

19

Vallejo

14

15

Presidio

Lover's Lane

Lyon Stwy.

Broadway

Divisadero

Scott

Pierce

Steiner

Presidio
Gate

Broadway
Gate

18

Pacific

17

16

Raycliff

PACIFIC HEIGHTS

QUICK-STEP INSTRUCTIONS

1. Begin your walk at the turn of the Presidio Wall on Lyon. Turn left on Gorgas. Left at four green posts into Letterman Digital Arts Center garden (unmarked Gorgas Gate).

2. Left and ascend stone stairway. Walk past metal arches by the pond.

3. Ascend the stone slab stairway and walk the paths, see the sculptures, explore the area, and return to the Gorgas Gate.

4. Descend stairway to Gorgas at Lyon. Turn right to the crosswalks.

5. Follow the crosswalks to the Palace of Fine Arts. Walk into the inner courtyard and rotunda, strolling among the ruins. Continue to the former Exploratorium.

6. At the former Exploratorium front parking area, bear right to the crosswalk on Marina Blvd.

7. Walk across and continue to the water. Right toward the St. Francis Yacht Club.

8. Continue to the Golden Gate Yacht Club and the jetty's end to the Wave Organ. Return to the Crissy Field entrance.

8a. *Optional:* Walk west along the water on the Coastal Trail into Crissy Field to Fort Point and the Golden Gate Bridge. Return to Crissy Field entrance.

9. Walk back to Marina Blvd. and Lyon. Cross the boulevard.

10. Left to Baker, and right on Baker.

11. Walk along the front of the Palace of Fine Arts and lagoon to Bay.

12. Left on Bay to Broderick.

13. Right on Broderick to Vallejo.

14. Left on Vallejo to Divisadero.

15. Right on Divisadero to Pacific.

16. Right on Pacific to Raycliff Terrace. Walk into cul-de-sac. Return to Pacific.

17. Right on Pacific to Lyon.

18. Right on Lyon. Descend Lyon Stairway.

19. Continue on Lyon to the end of the Presidio Wall and your beginning.

the largest lessee in the Presidio. Currently, the LDAC houses Lucas Arts and Industrial Light and Magic. The employees number around 1,300. Skywalker Sound, another branch, is situated in Marin County.

⌐ The LDAC was in process for five years from its design stage to the opening. The architects were Gensler Architecture & Design and HKS, Inc. It is on the site of the dismantled Letterman Army Hospital, from which 80% of the materials—cement, metals, and timber—were recycled and used in the LDAC's construction. The archaeology is so recent that it is still easy for me to visualize the area as it was.

◢ The Gen II Otis elevators in the buildings are the most efficient in use of energy. Raised flooring allows for ventilation in all the buildings. The windows are designed for the best circulation of air. The center stairwells are sunlit to encourage people to use the stairs. Many aspects of the buildings encourage conservation of energy. In addition the LDAC bought new materials from suppliers within a short radius of the Presidio to cut down on travel and fuel. For all of these reasons, the campus received a LEED Gold–certified rating from the Green Building Institute in 2006.

◢ Return to the Gorgas Gate, where you entered. A plaque on the top of the stairway states, "This site is managed and maintained by Letterman Digital Arts Ltd." Descend the stairway to Gorgas near Lyon. Veer to the right, and follow the crosswalks to your left, across Richardson, to the Palace of Fine Arts. At Bay, walk on the path into the inner courtyard and rotunda. Bernard Maybeck designed the Palace of Fine Arts, the only architectural survivor of the 1915 Panama-Pacific International Exposition. The building has been renovated by the funds raised through the Maybeck Foundation, the City of San Francisco, and private sources.

◢ Bear left around the theater toward the former Exploratorium, now relocated to the Embarcadero (see Walk 29). The Exploratorium is one of the city's most vital museums and a model for science museums throughout the world. It moved to its new home, occupying Piers 15 and 17, in 2013.

◢ At the former Exploratorium's front parking area, walk to the crosswalk at Marina Blvd. Cross the street and continue to the water. Turn right toward the St. Francis Yacht Club. At the end of the parking lot is an impressive Rolex Clock. Continue to the Golden Gate Yacht Club to reach the Wave Organ at the jetty's end. This wave-activated acoustic sculpture was designed by Peter Richards, and built by sculptor and master stonemason George Gonzalez, under the aegis of the Exploratorium. It is situated in the sound garden the artists designed, a terraced amphitheater built of recycled marble and granite acquired from a dismantled cemetery. The idea was to sit, enjoy the view of the skyline, and listen to the music as the pipes, which extend down into the Bay, respond to the movement of the water. The project was completed in spring of 1986, as part of the Exploratorium's science and art collection, and was dedicated to Frank Oppenheimer, the museum's founder.

◢ Return to the Crissy Field entrance. As an optional side trip, you may continue along the water onto the Coastal Trail to reach the restored Crissy Field, a 20-acre tidal marsh with a new shoreline promenade and restored beach and dunes. Here you can observe windsurfers and may even catch one of the regular windsurfing competitions. (Prior to 1915, the US Army used Crissy Field as a dump; in the 1920s, the space was used for an airfield and a rifle range.) You can continue on the trail to Fort Point, built in 1861 for defense against the South during the Civil War. Its walls are 7 feet thick and 45 feet high, and it survived the 1906 earthquake. Retrace your steps to the Crissy Field entrance.

Edward Payson Weston began a 500-mile walk from San Francisco to Los Angeles on May 25, 1908. People were invited to join him at any point and walk as far as they wanted. He left the Olympic Club on Post St. at 12 p.m. sharp and reached LA in 10 days.

◢ Turn right and walk back to the Marina Blvd. Cross the boulevard at the crosswalk, and turn left to Baker. At Baker turn right, walking along the front of the Palace of Fine Arts and the lagoon. The area around the lagoon is a popular place for people to picnic, sunbathe, and have their wedding parties photographed. In and around the lagoon, you will see swans, mallards, and night herons. When Adah was there, she identified a European widgeon, a bufflehead, and some coots. Turtles may be out on a sunny day, and sometimes you can see fish in the water.

◢ Turn left on Bay. Two murals in the 2300 block add a personal touch to the long block. Continue to Broderick, and then right on Broderick to walk uphill to Vallejo. The houses are eclectic and architecturally sound. No. 2821 Broderick and the house to the right, dating from about 1907, were the earliest on the block.

◢ The sidewalk on Broderick from Vallejo to Broadway is extremely steep and uncomfortable to climb, plus it is private property—bypass it. Instead, turn left on Vallejo to Divisadero. Turn right on Divisadero to Broadway. At Broadway look left for a spectacular view of the city's downtown. Continue to Pacific and turn right. At Pacific walk into Raycliff Terrace, a cul-de-sac of six houses designed by contemporary architects.

◢ Return to Pacific, and turn right and walk to Lyon. The El Drisco Hotel at 2901 Pacific (48 rooms) was built as a boardinghouse in 1903; it became a hotel in the 1930s. No. 2950 is a tuck-in, set in some distance from the sidewalk. An unusual variance gives three houses at No. 3070 one driveway with entrances on both Pacific and Lyon.

◢ At the intersection of Pacific and Lyon, you are 379 feet above sea level. This corner was named Cannon Hill for the symbolic cannon placed on the summit to mark the southeast corner of the Presidio (in the late 1870s). Turn right on Lyon to walk north along the Presidio Wall, enjoying a view of the Palace of Fine Arts' Romanesque rotunda, with the Marin hills as a backdrop.

◢ At Broadway descend the imposing Lyon Stairway—designed by Louis Upton in 1916—an arrangement of stairs, landings, and garden spaces. The Broadway neighbor to the right of the stairway has taken the initiative to renovate the gardens. The slope is covered with ivy. Surprisingly, it has a beautiful, undulating effect as you walk on the stairs. In spring, the blossoms on the plum trees and the colors and shapes of the annuals planted alongside the stairs draw you to them.

◢ On the ledge of the next set of stairs is a plaque dedicated to the memory of Ann Fogelberg, who spearheaded the Lyon St. Pride Project, a street cleanup and planting of trees project that introduced thousands of *Vinca major* plants to the slopes of the Lyon Stairway between

Lyon Stairway   *Adah Bakalinsky*

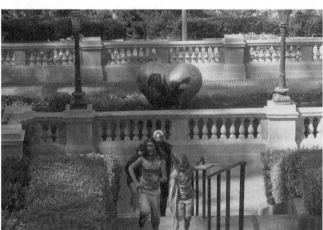

Vallejo and Green. Ann recruited neighborhood people and was able to enlist help from high school students and even organizations like the Department of Public Works Environmental Street Services agency and San Francisco Beautiful, among many others.

◢ The stairway ends in the cul-de-sac of Green. The six houses to your left, designed by architect August Headman and built in 1923, stand on part of the Miranda land grant, awarded to Juana Miranda (who had been married to Corporal A. Miranda of the Presidio). Under the oval center is the Agua de Figueroa spring, where the Presidio horses quenched their thirst, as do the successfully growing three redwoods and cypress trees.

◢ Continue on Lyon, past Lombard (looking back occasionally to view the homes on the heights) to the end of the Presidio Wall and back to your beginning.

Further Rambling

Chestnut St., the Marina's authentic and stable shopping area, is again thriving after the effects of the devastating 1989 earthquake. It's fun to be part of the ambling, strolling shoppers and greet friends you haven't seen since last week. The Presidio Theatre, just west down Chestnut at Scott St., plays current run movies and art films in the area, a nice respite after a brisk walk.

A Magical Walk

Fort Winfield Scott in the Presidio

We are fortunate, living in San Francisco, to enjoy within the city boundaries a legacy of 1,490 acres of open space, which was home to the Native American Ohlone tribe as far back as 3,000 years ago. Subsequently, the area became a Spanish military post (1776), a Mexican military post (1821), and then an American military post (1846–1994). In 1972, in one of its finest moments, Congress passed legislation creating the Golden Gate National Recreation Area (GGNRA). California Congressman Phillip Burton wrote this extraordinary law.

One of the stipulations of the GGNRA was that the Presidio, a US Army post, would become part of the National Park Service and the GGNRA, if the Army did not need it. The Department of the Interior, in 1982, designated the Presidio as a National Historic Landmark and officially recognized 500 historic buildings within it. In the fall of 1994, the transfer went into effect.

Because the Presidio is so vast, has approximately 800 buildings, and will eventually have more than 50 miles of trails and eight scenic overlooks available for visitors to enjoy, the cost of maintaining such a wealth of natural and human-made resources is high. Therefore, in 1996, Congress created a new federal agency, the Presidio Trust to manage the noncoastal areas of the Presidio (1,192 acres). The Presidio Trust supervises and leases the residential and commercial properties.

Meanwhile, much good work is being done to promote the historical preservation and the natural diversity of the area. Some of the projects include developing habitat to increase the population of 200 species of birds year-round, including migratory and resident varieties; replacing eucalyptus trees that have reached their 100-year maturity with native trees; and restoring Lobos Creek, the water source for the Presidio. It's impressive to witness the dedication of the staff and volunteers, and the direction the Presidio is taking in working with open space, the scenic views, and native plant areas.

There are 1,109 units in the Presidio available for housing. The housing is leased at market prices except for a few accommodations for resident rangers and park police. Some units have been set aside for low-cost housing.

The western section of the Presidio is known as Fort Winfield Scott. In 1912, the Coast Artillery Group was formed to protect the coast. It was and still is part of the Presidio, but it was given its own fort, named after the general.

When you begin a walk, it's best to begin it as a stroll. You don't know what you are looking for, but suddenly, something feels appealing. This walk's appeal is in the series of river-washed rocks fashioned into very long, low retaining walls along Kobbe Ave., the street lined with officers' homes. Soon the river-rock wall supports run along stairways, leading farther on to woodsy paths among random rows of eucalyptus trees and Monterey pines. Walking down the stairways here, and stepping into the leafy, overgrown areas, you can feel how the atmosphere changes in the windy mist. It has a primeval quality and a feeling of mystery that enhances the stroll, making you eager to continue.

WALK FACTS

The Presidio Trust offers a free monthly shuttle tour, limited to four people per party. Call ahead for reservations and to get a preview of the multiple forts once located in San Francisco; stops include the Main Post, Fort Scott, Crissy Field, and the coastal bluffs. For reservations, call 415-561-5418 or e-mail **presidio@presidiotrust.gov**.

Presidio Park Stewards and Shoreline Maintenance volunteer crews gather monthly to replant native plants and preserve habitat in the city's wildlife corridors.

Bus Routes & Parking

PUBLIC TRANSPORTATION: MUNI Bus #28 19th Ave. and #29 Sunset; free PresidiGo Shuttle. For MUNI bus information, call 311 (outside San Francisco, call 415-701-2311). For PresidiGo Shuttle information, call the Trust Transportation Department at 415-561-5300 or visit **presidigo.gov**.

PARKING: Park in the lot across from Barnard Hall, 1330 Kobbe, or use the free PresidiGo Park Shuttles. PresidiGo runs every 30 minutes seven

(Continued on page 88)

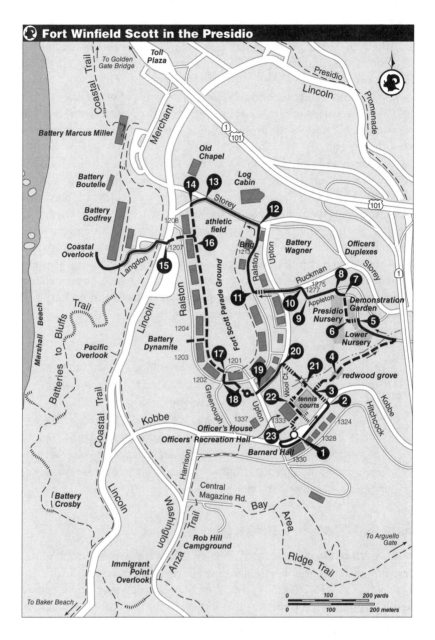

Fort Winfield Scott in the Presidio

QUICK-STEP INSTRUCTIONS

1. Cross Kobbe at the corner of Upton. Turn left toward No. 1324. Cross Kobbe at the crosswalk.

2. Descend stairway, and continue ahead on walkway.

3. Right to descend second set of stairs. Continue to the open space.

4. Walk to the right through the redwood grove and down right side of seasonal creek to the lower area of Presidio Nursery and demonstration garden on hillsides. Turn left.

5. Bear left to ascend peeler-core stairway to the upper portion of the Presidio Nursery.

6. Right past greenhouses.

7. Left between buildings and parking area.

8. Left on Appleton at No. 1275.

9. Right at No. 1277 to Ruckman.

10. Left on Ruckman and walk on left side. Ascend the sidewalk stairways to Ralston.

11. Right on Ralston past the Brig to Storey.

12. Left on Storey (detour to look at Log Cabin across the street). Continue on Storey.

13. Bear left on the first street (around baseball field) to No. 1208.

14. Left at No. 1208 onto the Ft. Scott Walkway.

15. Right between Nos. 1208 and 1207, and cross Lincoln Blvd. at Langdon Court. Follow Bay Area Ridge Trail sign to Battery Godfrey. Explore and return to No. 1208.

16. Right at No. 1207, following the Ridge Trail to No. 1204. Turn right to walk between Nos. 1204 and 1203 to look at Battery Dynamite. Explore and return to No. 1203. Continue to No. 1202.

17. Right to Ralston.

18. Left on Ralston and walk on an old concrete path that crosses the lawn at the corner of Ralston and Upton.

19. Continue straight ahead and then downhill on Upton to its intersection with Wool Court.

20. At the intersection street sign, descend stone stairways, cross bridge, and ascend stairway.

21. Right at first path. Walk along tennis courts up to a paved parking area.

22. Left and walk alongside the curved window wall of the Officers' Recreation Hall, No. 1333.

23. Right, at end of the building, to ascend the curved stairway to the parking lot across from No. 1330 Kobbe, and your beginning.

(Continued from page 85)

days a week (Monday–Friday, 6:30 a.m.–7:30 p.m.; Saturday, Sunday, and holidays, 11 a.m.–6 p.m.).

NOTE: Pick up a free PresidiGo schedule and map of the area at the Presidio Visitors' Center in the Old Officers club at No. 50 Moraga (the entrance is notable for a nearby cannon). You can also call 415-561-4323 and request that the information be mailed to you. Take the circle tour to become familiar with the general layout of the park.

WALK 9 DESCRIPTION

◢ Park across the street from Barnard Hall, 1330 Kobbe St., the building known as BOQ (Bachelor Officers' Quarters). The residences along this street were formerly used for officers and their families. At the Upton intersection, cross Kobbe. Walk left to No. 1324 (three houses down), built in 1912. In 1883 Major William A. Jones submitted a plan for introducing trees to the Presidio. Acacia, pine, eucalyptus, native redwood, madrone, spruce, and palm were planted in the 1880s and 1890s, many of them by schoolchildren on Arbor Day. Cross Kobbe at the crosswalk, opposite No. 1324. Descend the concrete stairway with sidewalls of river rock. Part of the walkway is brick.

◢ After many years of neglect, the forest is being rehabilitated. The walk here has improved from a setting of neglect with broken, dying trees and overgrown masses of ivy and mattress wire weed (*Muehlenbeckia*), to an area of wholly optimum conditions. Here now are areas cleared of ivy, and the introduction of native plantings as well. These improvements provide food for birds and wildlife, and allow for happy, healthy trees and shrubs to grow. Continue down the stairs and next to the tennis courts, and turn right to descend another small set of stairs to a footpath. The footpath leads a few feet farther on, to open space. (In all, the Presidio YMCA manages six tennis courts, located throughout the Presidio; check their website for further details.)

◢ Continue toward the right, through a redwood grove, downward on the footpath, which is considered a social trail because it was created by walkers and not the Park Service. Follow along the right side of Dragonfly Creek, which, though always damp, is relatively dry in fall and wet in the winter. Farther on, past the nursery, the creek culverts down toward Crissy Field. On your left, lying helter-skelter on the ground, is a collection of granite slabs with incised names, rubble left from the 1906 earthquake. These historic slabs were originally stored at Lands End, but they were brought to the Presidio because people were removing them for their personal collections. In front of you is the lower section of the Presidio Nursery, shade houses are open and allow for climate control. The Park Conservancy, a nonprofit group, manages the test planting and restoration work with a staff of two full-time horticulturalists, complemented by interns and volunteers. Participants are welcome to assist on Wednesdays and Saturdays from 1 p.m. to 4 p.m. The Presidio Nursery is the largest nursery in the entire GGNRA; seedlings for Crissy Field are grown here.

◢ Turn left to note the flagged demonstration garden along the hillside on both sides. The garden showcases the various habitats that occur in the Presidio, from oak woodland to sandy dunes to serpentine grassland. Turn left at the small bridge, and ascend the peeler-core stairway to the upper Presidio Nursery. The nursery is clean of debris and so well organized, with containers of young plants in alphabetical order, ready to be dispersed according to plan, that you feel as if you can come in for the first time and know where to find exactly what you need. The nursery area has undergone renovations, including the construction of a wetland area and offers outreach work and ongoing volunteer activities.

◢ Children five years or older, as well as adults, are welcome and encouraged to participate in the Presidio Nursery program, which offers teaching tools suitable for grades six through eight. Summer camp is also available. Planting in the rain, when the soil is at optimum consistency and the process feels like finger painting, is enjoyed by class groups on a grand scale in the spring. A permanent Center for Sustainability opened in 2010, adding classrooms and labs, as well as kitchen and bathroom facilities that can accommodate larger numbers of students and adults.

◢ To the right of the stairway are greenhouses with native plant seedlings. Walk past the greenhouses, and veer left between the buildings and parking lot. Walk to an unmarked street, Appleton. You will see the sign for No. 1275 across the street. Turn left and walk past the row of enlisted-family housing on the right that has been renovated for leasing with a view of downtown San Francisco behind you.

◢ Turn right at No. 1277 to Ruckman, then left. Walk on the left side, pass Upton, and ascend short sidewalk stairways to Ralston. Turn right and pass the Brig, a flat-roofed, two-story building. You might think that it once offered its inmates the best views. It would have if the windows were at eye level, but the second-story floor is so low that you would need a ladder to see out of the window. Many windows on the other buildings have bars across them, which were added for protection in case someone accidentally forgot to close them.

◢ Continue on Ralston to Storey. The Log Cabin straight ahead was built of timber logs and rock in 1937 by the Works Progress Administration. The interior has wagon wheel chandeliers, a huge fireplace, space for large groups to dine or dance, and a view of the meadow and San Francisco. (For rental information, call 415-561-5444.) Go left on Storey, then bear left on the first street around the softball field to No. 1208. Turn left at 1208 to continue on the Fort Scott Walkway. Turn right between Nos. 1208 and 1207.

◢ Cross Lincoln Blvd. at the Langdon Court crosswalk, to follow a small section of the Bay Area Ridge Trail. (Watch for cars.) Follow the trail sign to Battery Godfrey and explore the area a bit. An interpretive sign gives some of its history. On a very clear day, you can look out from here and see the Farallon Islands; when it happens, it's quite a moment! But weather here normally is overcast, and the islands remain hidden. However, from this viewpoint, you can also see the curve of the span of the Golden Gate Bridge. You can walk across the bridge and drive across it, but it's hard to feel the curve. The Fort Scott viewpoint adds another dimension to your perspective of the bridge, as you can become more familiar with an object by knowing it from multiple angles. (For more bridge view locations, see Further Rambling at the end of this walk.)

◢ Return to the Fort Scott Walkway. Cross Lincoln Blvd. at the crosswalk. At the side of No. 1208, looking toward the green meadow, you see the Bay Bridge, which Adah calls the Cinderella Bridge—by day, it is a working bridge; by night, it becomes a sparkling phantom bridge, enveloped by glittering lights. (A friend suggested the "Two Bridge Walk" as a subtitle.) You also see Coit Tower and Russian Hill. Continue walking alongside the enlisted men's barracks, which are built of concrete and stucco, in the Mission Revival style. Italian stone pines, which reach maturity after 50 to 70 years, have been planted along the row. The pine in front of No. 1206 is striking, with large galls surrounding the trunk. (Galls are part of the tree, and not a disease.)

◢ Turn right to walk back between Nos. 1204 and 1203, and go into Battery Dynamite if the gate is open. What you see first is a 40-foot

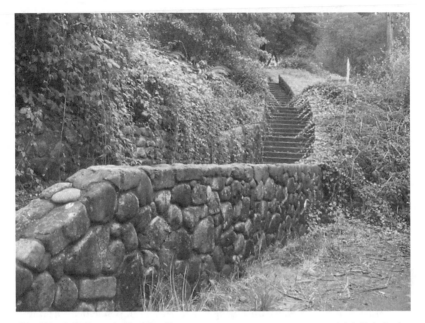

River Rock Stairway in Fort Scott   *Adah Bakalinsky*

wall. There is a series of tunnels underneath, with three gun pits used for testing dynamite weapons during the 1890s. The problem of how to light the fuse without causing an explosion was solved by using the small, hidden Greek-style structure to the right of the wall as an air compressor for the new dynamite test guns, which operated like huge air compression rifles. The tests were successful. The shells could land in the water near a ship, and the concussion would break the hull. There was one problem: the short range of 2 miles. Since other coast-defense guns with a longer range were being developed, the dynamite test weapon was laid to rest.

"Well, here we go, up the apple and pears." This Cockney expression from the east end of London means, "Here we go, up the stairs."

⊿ Return to the Parade Ground and continue to No. 1202 to read the interpretive sign for Fort Winfield Scott. Turn right and continue to Ralston. Turn left and walk on the concrete path that crosses the lawn at the corner of Ralston and Upton. The area must have been a garden at some earlier time.

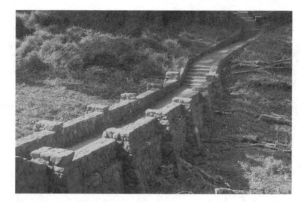

Upton at Wool Court   *Tony Holiday*

◢ Continue straight ahead, down Upton to its intersection with Wool Court. At the intersection street sign, descend the stone stairways, and walk across the stone bridge. The slopes have been cleared and planted. Along this trail you can see perchance, as Adah spied once, Oregon juncos and spotted towhees. Continue to ascend the stairway.

◢ At the first path, turn right beside the tennis courts. Turn left alongside the curved window wall of the Officers' Recreation Hall, No. 1331. Turn right at the end of the building, and ascend the curved stairway to your beginning.

Further Rambling

Opposite Battery Godfrey, at the edge of the trees, a sign notes, "Baker Beach and Batteries to Bluffs Trail." This path leads to multiple stairways, ascending and descending, along the bluffs of the Pacific Ocean to Battery Chamberlain at Baker Beach. If you want to continue, cross Lincoln Blvd. and ascend the connector stairway to Immigrant Point Overlook and the Rob Hill Campground. You can return on the same route or walk the Coastal Trail along Lincoln Blvd. back to Langdon.

　　Another option: Take PresidiGo to Stop 31 to enjoy the view at the San Francisco National Cemetery Overlook, slightly northeast of Fort Scott. The overlook provides contemplative views of the cemetery and San Francisco Bay. It was first dedicated on Veterans Day in 2009, and the slabs display the poem "Young Dead Soldiers" by Archibald MacLeish, who served in World War I.

Sutro's Legacy for All Time

Lands End

Each visit to Lands End seems to improve upon the next because the area is still actively being restored. Thanks to the now-defunct Richard and Rhoda Goldman Fund, donations totaling $9 million were made to this restoration project, making the fund its lead supporter. The work of the restoration project has brought us graceful paved footpaths, new views of the Bay, comfortable redwood stairways, and attractively designed direction signs. We have the opportunity to awaken our senses and take in the colors and sounds of a wilderness area briskly surrounded by wind, ocean, and the Bay, and yet we are within the city.

From Point Lobos Ave. and El Camino del Mar, we are in an area of the city known as the Sutro District, named for San Francisco hero Adolph Sutro. The majority of wealthy citizens in the late 1800s settled in the Nob Hill, Rincon Hill, and South Park neighborhoods. Sutro settled and developed the northwest part of the city, which he loved for its beauty, fog, and ocean air. As it evolved, he understood its potential as open space and parkland with opportunities for recreation that families could enjoy.

Sutro came to the United States in 1850 from Aix-la-Chapelle (Aachen), Germany, with his mother and seven siblings. He was 20 years old, had a high school education, worked in the family cloth factory, read voraciously, and was self-taught in mining and engineering.

Using the profits he accrued from the sale of his shares in his first large engineering project in the United States, the 4-mile-long tunnel built to drain and ventilate the Nevada Comstock silver mines, Sutro developed and designed the Sutro Baths, an elaborate arrangement of pools with varying temperatures to be enjoyed by families. He built the Sutro Railroad to provide low-cost (5¢) transportation for family outings—swimming in the Sutro Baths, dining at the Cliff House, or walking on the grounds of his 21-acre Sutro Heights Estate of sculpture and landscaped gardens.

Sutro planted eucalyptus trees to hold the soil of the sand dunes (while his choice of species was not native to San Francisco, they hold the soil). He founded the Sutro Library and even opened his private property

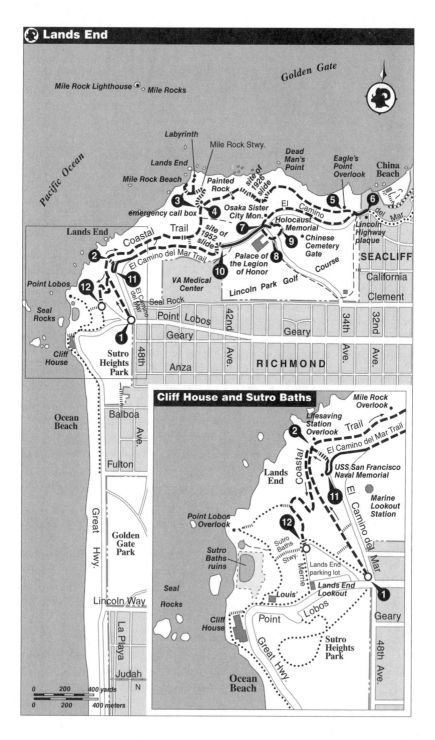

QUICK-STEP INSTRUCTIONS

1. Begin at El Camino del Mar and Point Lobos Ave. at the Sutro District sign. Walk on the right paved footpath past stairways to the interpretive sign.

2. Continue veering right on the Coastal Trail. Pass the stairway leading to the USS *San Francisco Naval Memorial,* and continue past retaining walls. Descend a log stairway, and pass another stairway on the right. Turn left at the junction.

3. At the Mile Rock Beach sign, descend the Mile Rock Stairway to the beach and Labyrinth at Lands End.

4. Return to the Coastal Trail. Turn left and pass Painted Rock. Ascend the long stairway, and descend other shorter stairways.

5. At the stairways, Dead Man's Point is on your left. Continue to Eagle's Point Platform.

6. Continue on the Coastal Trail to El Camino del Mar into Seacliff. Right on 32nd Ave. to view Lincoln Highway post.

7. Return to El Camino del Mar (at 32nd Ave.), continue on the right side of the road toward the Palace of the Legion of Honor, and turn left.

8. Walk to the museum. Across the road at the bus stop is the Lincoln Highway plaque.

9. Walk past the pool to the *Holocaust Memorial.* Turn left to walk past the *Osaka Sister City Monument.*

10. Walk through the parking area. Descend the wood stairway to El Camino del Mar Trail. It leads to a dirt path and boardwalk. Continue on the trail to the naval memorial.

11. To the right of the memorial, descend the stairway to the Coastal Trail and turn left.

12. At a fork in the road, veer right. Continue toward the Merrie Way (Lands End) parking lot. Turn left and continue to your beginning.

to the general public. He was mayor from 1894 to 1896 and died in 1898. Sutro left San Francisco a profound and beneficent legacy. Sutro Heights, the Sutro Baths ruins, and the Cliff House are all now under the jurisdiction of the Golden Gate National Recreation Area.

WALK FACTS

Wind, rain, or shine, Lands End offers walkers beautiful ocean views during the day, stargazing at night, and fabulous sunsets in between. If you walk around the grounds of Sutro's mansion, remember to leave at dusk.

The Sutro Egyptian collection is now mostly housed at San Francisco State University, but some pieces are on loan to the Cliff House. Stop in to see early bathing suits, bathhouse posters, and admission tickets in the restaurant and bar.

Behind the Cliff House, visit the Camera Obscura and Holograph Gallery. The Camera Obscura is last remaining structure from Playland, and it opened in 1946. The outside was fashioned to look like a camera in the 1950s. Take the stairs behind the Cliff House down to the exhibit (open until around dusk).

Bus Routes & Parking

PUBLIC TRANSPORTATION: MUNI Bus #18 46th Avenue, #31 Balboa St., and #38 Geary stops at 48th and Point Lobos. Walk two blocks west. For MUNI bus information, call 311 (outside San Francisco, call 415-701-2311).

PARKING: You can park at two different parking lots near Lands End on Point Lobos. Geary becomes Point Lobos when it crosses 48th Avenue. Parking is available for the *War Memorial* and for Sutro Heights Park. There is also free and metered street parking available, usually allowed for up to one and two hours, respectively. But also look for street-cleaning times posted in the neighborhood to avoid getting ticketed or towed.

WALK 10 DESCRIPTION

Begin your walk at El Camino del Mar and Point Lobos Ave. at the Sutro District GGNRA sign. Walk on the right paved footpath 0.3 mile to the Coastal Trail. Lawrence Halprin, the landscape architect whose work we will be viewing as we continue our walk, was well known for his attention to greening within the context of the urban environment. The succulents and native plants that accompany this walk feel like the perfect solution for the setting. The plants are tended and planted by large groups of volunteers. (If you are interested in this work, call the Presidio Trust at 415-561-5333 to volunteer.) Along the paths, look for native plants, such as sticky monkeyflower, lupines, and California poppies. The multitude of little yellow flowers, sorrel on long stems, that abound along the footpaths are beautiful, but they are weeds and will take over an area. The National Parks Conservancy

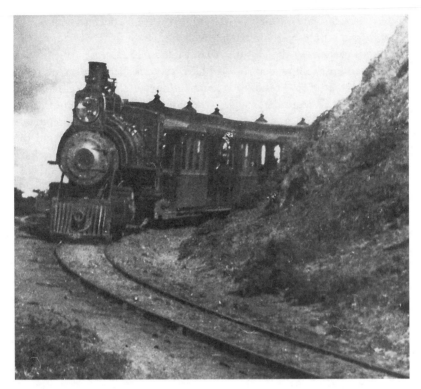

Sutro Railroad, ca. 1890   *Courtesy of National Park Service*

and National Park Service are doing their best to eradicate them. The brush sculpture, made from cut tree refuse, is a haven for birds. You can often hear white crown sparrows circling around it.

⊿ Walk past the two stairways to the interpretive sign. Continue veering right and walk past the stairway leading to the USS *San Francisco Naval Memorial.*

⊿ You may soon hear foghorns. Their sounds may be coming from the Golden Gate Bridge, Point Bonita Lighthouse, or Mile Rock (a mile from the middle of the shipping channel, not a mile from shore). Each foghorn has a recognizable pattern of timed seconds of sound followed by timed seconds of silence. From the right side of the trail, you may periodically hear the gurgling sound of water, indicating a seep. Usually, you'll find a patch of green or flowers nearby, but watch out for poison oak.

◢ As you continue on the Coastal Trail, you see a concrete wall on the right side. Built as the retaining wall for the Sutro Railroad, it continues to support the hillside. A landslide in 1925 closed off most of the rail lines. Shipwreck spotters liked to come here via the railroad, which came from Presidio Ave. and California along the cliffs. Most shipwrecks occurred through some combination of fog, northwest winds, sand bars, and rocky shoals. At low tide you can see remnants of an engine block from the wreck of the *Lyman Stewart* and the sternpost of the *Frank Buck*. The next retaining walls and overlook offer the best views of them. During World War II, the US Army had coastal defenses and gun batteries along the cliff line here and spotting stations at Sutro Heights.

◢ Continue on the unpaved footpath, descend a short log stairway, and pass a stairway on your right that leads to El Camino del Mar Trail. This area has suffered landslides during heavy winter rains, and parts of the trail may be closed. Walk on any alternate path as indicated.

◢ Walk past some serpentine and granite rocks. When the path ends, continue left to the "Mile Rock Beach" sign and stairway. The Mile Rock Stairway is well built and comfortable to walk, and it leads you to the ocean, where waves continually crash against the huge rocks. Ascend the path to the right to see the Labyrinth, constructed in the

Post commemorating the Lincoln Highway

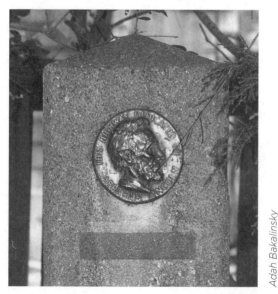

Adah Bakalinsky

sand at the point of Lands End by Eduardo Aguilera. Walk it and solve it, but you may find that the weather is trying to reclaim it. Nude beaches are nearby. The return up the stairway is moderately difficult. If you prefer to omit it, continue on the Coastal Trail. Painted Rock on your right was a US Coast Guard navigational tool used as a sight line with Point Bonita Lighthouse in the Marin Headlands.

◢ Just ahead in the fenced area on your left (a warning sign at Painted Rock cliff) was the tunnel through which Sutro's train rounded the bend. The tunnel collapsed, the cliff partially fell away, and the trail was rerouted uphill and around to the right.

◢ Ascend the long stairway, and curve left to descend shorter stairways. You will pass Dead Man's Point on the left, and then reach Eagle's Point Platform, which you can ascend via a ramp or stairway. As you walk across the platform, you have the opportunity to savor slightly varied views of Seacliff, China Beach, Baker Beach, the Golden Gate Bridge, and Fort Point. Return to the path.

◢ Turn left and walk to the end of the trail. Cross El Camino del Mar, and turn left to 32nd Ave. On the left side of 32nd Ave. is a commemorative post for the Lincoln Highway, the first transcontinental highway, which was built in 1915. It extended from Times Square in New York City to Lincoln Park in San Francisco. Retrace your steps and turn right into the Seacliff neighborhood. Seacliff was developed in 1924, with curving streets and gateway entrances at 25th, 26th, and 27th Aves. The homes are large, the ocean views from north-facing windows are vivid, and the gardens on the south side are verdant.

◢ Mark Daniels, former general superintendent and landscape engineer of the National Park Service, laid out the system of curving streets and terraces. (He also designed the street pattern in Forest Hill, Walk 15.) The architect Willis Polk designed three homes in Seacliff—Nos. 9, 25, and 45 Scenic Way.

◢ Recollecting his childhood, a former resident of Seacliff remembers walking through the sand dunes and the seas of gold and purple lupine. Rabbits, snakes, and wild canaries lived in the area then; he remembers his father trapping the canaries and feeding them hard-boiled eggs. He also recalls fishing every other day from Lands End.

◢ When you are ready to begin the return route, go back to El Camino del Mar (at 32nd Ave.), and walk on the right side toward the Palace of the Legion of Honor. Continue walking past 17 memorial benches and the *World Peace Monument* along the way. Views of the Bay are to the right. The path borders the Lincoln Park Golf Course. At the *Holocaust Memorial,* turn left to the Palace of the Legion of Honor. If you wish to see the current exhibit and have lunch in the museum, go in (members get in free, but other visitors must pay an entry fee).

◢ On the knoll of the Lincoln Park Golf Course are some of the remnants of the 1868 cemetery. More than 1,000 graves, many of them Chinese, were discovered when the museum was retrofitted and redesigned in 1993. To see the one remaining Chinese cemetery gate, walk down the Legion of Honor Drive for about 0.1 mile. The gate will be on your left, in the middle of the golf course, easily seen embedded between two cypress trees. (Do not walk onto the golf course.)

◢ Across from the museum at the bus stop is a plaque that reads, "This highway dedicated to Abraham Lincoln." It's a replacement of the original one that disappeared. Three sides of the post display replicas of Lincoln's face.

◢ Walk toward the pool to see the outdoor sculptures: Closest to the pool is *Pax Jerusalem* by Mark di Suvero, a large orange abstract. The *Holocaust Memorial* by George Segal is to the left of the pool. To get the full emotional impact of the sculpture, view it from the platform. Toward the left is the *Osaka Sister City Monument.*

◢ Turn left beyond the monument along the paved parking area. Descend the wood stairway onto the El Camino del Mar Trail. Continue walking on the path past the stairway to the Coastal Trail. The building seen above to your left is the VA Medical Center.

◢ The path leads to the parking lot on El Camino del Mar where the USS *San Francisco Naval Memorial* is located. The memorial was formed from the bridge of the ship after it was torpedoed in November 1942 during the Battle of Guadalcanal.

◢ In this area, there once existed a series of signal stations, where people were stationed to spot different ships coming in through the Golden Gate. They would then relay the information, originally via semaphores and later via telegraph, to the wharf area. One relay station structure, the Octagon House, remains above the parking lot, up toward the trees on the left. A semaphore attached to it was used to relay a particular ship's arrival to Telegraph Hill and Fisherman's Wharf. When electricity became available, the telegraph replaced the semaphores.

◢ Descend the stairway to the right of the memorial to the Coastal Trail, and turn left. At the fork in the road, veer right. Along the path is a continuation of the new native plantings of the coastal dunes. Before you reach the stairway into Merrie Way (Lands End) parking lot, turn left to your beginning.

Further Rambling

In the days when the Sutro Baths were operating, Adolph Sutro installed amusement rides where the Merrie Way (Lands End) parking lot is located. Interpretive signs are near the walkway. From there, descend the stairway to the Sutro Baths ruins. The baths were opened in 1896 and closed in 1952, and the buildings were destroyed by fire in 1966. In this eroded sandstone setting, with the offshore Seal Rocks in the background, are broken columns, fragments of tile mosaic, and the emptied pool area extending toward the ocean. The sea lions, formerly at home on Hermit Rock, moved to Pier 39 in 1989 for a reason that remains unknown—perhaps as a result of the Loma Prieta earthquake or some other natural phenomenon. (As early explorers approached from the ocean side a distance away, Angel and Alcatraz Islands looked like a continuous horizon line rather than islands in a bay. This explains why San Francisco was discovered via a land route from the south, rather than from the sea.)

In 1865 James Cooke walked from the Cliff House to Seal Rocks on a tightrope.

Bear right to the Point Lobos Overlook. The view of the Pacific Ocean and the Marin Headlands from here is mesmerizing. When you're ready to continue, walk on the curving path toward the right among the ruins. As you explore the area, follow the designated paths. You are allowed to enter the open tunnel that Sutro dug during the construction of the baths. The inside path can be slippery. To your left are the former pools, one of freshwater, the others salt. The honeycomb rectangle was the heating plant. Adolph Sutro designed and engineered the structure with its seven indoor pools, each heated to a different temperature. A swim, rental of a suit, towels, and a locker cost 25¢. There was room for 10,000 swimmers and seats for 7,000 spectators. The conservatories were decorated with palm trees and Egyptian artifacts.

Return on the path, and walk past the Sutro Baths Stairway. Primrose, lupine, poison oak, blackberry, and nasturtium grow alongside the path. You can also see dune tansy, blue bush lupine, beach primrose, and coyote bush. Park botanists are cultivating plants native to the area.

Albizia, the tall shrub with white spiky flowers, grows everywhere. It's beautiful, but invasive.

Ascend the incline toward Louis' Restaurant on Point Lobos Ave. To the right is the remodeled Cliff House. In addition to the two restaurants, you are welcome to view historical photos of Sutro Baths, Sutro Heights, and the Cliff House. If you want to explore the famous grounds of Sutro's home, walk to the arterial stop to cross Point Lobos Ave. This area is rich for exploring in all directions.

Another ambling jaunt takes you to the hiking paths along the Great Highway south of Balboa that have been tastefully landscaped for hikers and cyclists (sand control is more successful now than it used to be).

If you would like to explore China Beach to the east, continue on El Camino del Mar to Seacliff Ave. and China Beach. A stone placed at the top of the China Beach Stairway commemorates the Chinese fishermen who used this site. If you would like to continue farther to Baker Beach, follow the sign at No. 320 El Camino del Mar that reads "Public Beach." Turn left on Seacliff, and at 25th Ave. turn left into the cul-de-sac to take the stairway to Baker Beach.

MUNI Bus #29 and the PresidiGo Bus stop near Baker Beach. For a full day's outing, continue on El Camino del Mar to the Presidio, take Lincoln Blvd. to Fort Point, and continue on waterfront paths around Fisherman's Wharf and down the Embarcadero and the Blue Greenway (see Walks 6, 8, 9, and 29). With almost 4,000 acres of the GGNRA within the city, the walking opportunities are boundless!

Lead Thread on a Sugar Sack

Golden Gate Heights

Golden Gate Heights is one of the Sunset neighborhoods. Adah explained to me how scouting out this walk initially was reminiscent of trying to find the beginning loop thread on a 10-pound sugar sack. With one pull, she automatically unlocked the other loops. She described her discovery of the "lead stairway" in Golden Gate Heights as a path that magically "unlocked" all the other stairways in the neighborhood. This walk's uninterrupted, rhythmic line with its many curves undulating you forward will make you feel as if you are walking along with Matisse, painting the steps ahead of you.

When the Moraga Stairway was tiled back in 2004, Adah changed the order of this walk to have people ascend it rather than descend it, as it was designed in earlier editions. This way, walkers would enjoy viewing the tiles all the way up. But now a second tile work stairway installation, the Hidden Garden Steps, at 16th Avenue and Lawton down to Kirkham (see Further Rambling below to connect to it from this walk) once again offers readers the element of surprise. When adventurous walkers extend this walk, they will see that beauty lies at the end of the stairway, as well as its beginning.

The vast tract of land known as the Sunset District sprawls south from Golden Gate Park to Sloat Blvd. and from Stanyan to the Pacific Ocean. At one time it was all sand dunes, and a Sunday's outing to the beach with lunch or dinner at the Cliff House on the Great Highway was a gala occasion. Silting is a continual problem, but it has been minimized on the Great Highway by a design of raised paths for bicyclists and pedestrians, plus the planting of dune tansy and ice plant. The Outer Sunset is subject to magnificent sunsets, the ocean view, clean air, and wind and fog. The establishment of Golden Gate Park in 1870 promoted the settlement of

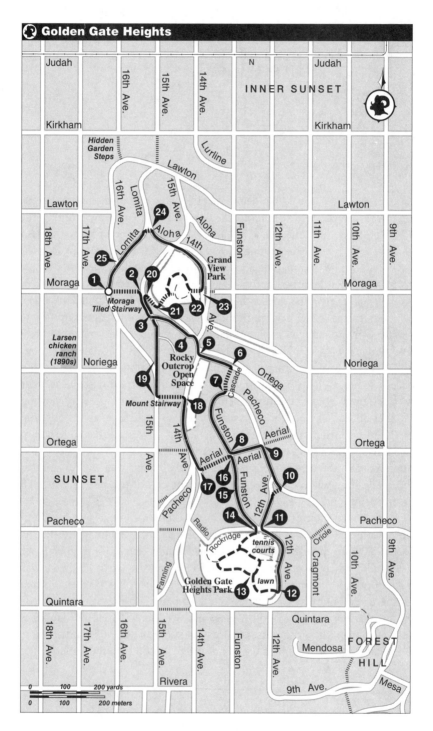

Golden Gate Heights

QUICK-STEP INSTRUCTIONS

1. Begin at Moraga and 16th Ave. Ascend tiled stairway to 15th Ave.
2. Right on 15th Ave to Noriega.
3. Left on Noriega to 14th Ave.
4. Right on 14th Ave. to Ortega.
5. Left on upper Ortega to Cascade Stairway.
6. Right and ascend to intersection of Funston and Pacheco.
7. Right on Funston to Aerial.
8. Left on Aerial to Pacheco.
9. Right on Pacheco to the triangular piece of land at 12th Ave.
10. Ascend curved stairway to 12th Ave.
11. Left on 12th Ave. to intersection of Rockridge and Cragmont across from Golden Gate Heights Park.
12. Cross the street and turn left to walk on the sidewalk. At No. 2026 cross the street and enter park on paved path. Walk through playground and turn left.
13. Follow this path to the roundabout and sitting area at the top of the park. Continue on path around north side. Turn left at tennis courts and walk to Rockridge.
14. Cross Rockridge to Funston.
15. Continue on Funston to Aerial Stairway.
16. Descend Aerial Stairway to 14th Ave.
17. Right on 14th Ave. to Mount Stairway.
18. Descend Mount Stairway (next to No. 1795 14th Ave.) to 15th Ave.
19. Right on 15th Ave. past Noriega to stairway at retaining wall.
20. Ascend stairway. Cross upper 15th Ave.
21. Ascend stairway to Grand View Park.
22. Walk left on sand footpath at second bench around park. On opposite side of park, descend stairway to 14th Ave.
23. Left on 14th Ave. to intersection of 14th Ave., 15th Ave., and Aloha.
24. Veer left on Aloha to corner stairway onto Lomita.
25. Continue left on Lomita to 16th Ave. Veer left to your beginning.

the Sunset. Other events continued the process: A railroad was built along H Street (Lincoln Way) to the beach in 1879; in 1898, the University of California Medical School was established; in 1904, a Midwinter Fair was held in Golden Gate Park; and in 1905, St. Anne's Church was founded. The 1906 earthquake brought people to the outer lands, away from the damaged areas of Telegraph Hill, North Beach, and Russian Hill.

The area's three leading contractors and builders in the Sunset: Henry Doelger, Raymond Galli, and Fred Gellert, used mass housing techniques (perfected in the 1920s). The new process enabled them to sell homes in the late 1930s for $5,000. Construction recommenced in 1945 after the end of World War II. Development of homes with tunnel entrances, the "Sunset look," where living rooms were built above garages, solved problems posed by smaller (25-foot by 65-foot) lots and the low $6,000 ceiling of available Federal Housing Administration loans. Between 60 and 80% of the homes are owner-occupied.

The Inner Sunset has a stable population of middle-class families of various ethnic origins. According to a 2008 report, Asians comprise 48.5%, Whites 44.9%, African Americans 1.33%, and Hispanics 4.5% (with the remaining 0.77% lumped into "Other").

WALK FACTS

Lovers of Carnegie library architecture can visit the Golden Gate Heights branch at 18th Ave. and Irving and enjoy one in person. More than 1,600 were built in the United States between 1883 and 1929; Andrew Carnegie believed that everybody should have the opportunity to improve themselves. Some sources even say that Carnegie associated staircases with elevated learning.

Grand View Park can get very windy, but it's worth visiting for an extended amount of time to take in a sunset.

Bus Routes & Parking

PUBLIC TRANSPORTATION: MUNI Bus #66 Quintara; #28 19th Ave.; and Metro N Judah. For MUNI bus or Metro information, call 311 (outside San Francisco, call 415-701-2311).

PARKING: There is metered street parking available; metered parking is usually available for up to an hour, and free street parking usually allowed for up to two hours. But also look for street-cleaning times posted in the neighborhood to avoid getting ticketed or towed.

WALK 11 DESCRIPTION

◢ Begin the walk by ascending the mosaic tile stairway at 16th Ave. and Moraga, which children call "the magic stairway." It is another fine example of the united community action that occurs in San Francisco.

A young woman who once lived in Rio de Janeiro and saw the Santa Teresa decorative stairway from her apartment window thought it would be wonderful if the concrete stairway she saw from her San Francisco window sang with colors instead of being a nondescript gray. She began talking with neighbors, found a kindred spirit living next door to the stairway who wholeheartedly endorsed the project, and volunteered her garage (and her wonderful baking skills) for neighborhood meetings and presentations of possible stairway designs by artists. Discussions with City officials of plans and fees; talks with possible donors of tile, paints, and equipment; and consultations regarding fundraising ideas and events ensued over a period of three years.

People now come from afar to see and walk the stairway. Busloads of senior citizens, schoolchildren, and preschool tots and their parents—all are entranced by the colorful mosaic tile stairway that tells a story of sky and water and birds and fish and flowers and frogs. On August 27, 2005, the newly designed stairway by local mosaic artists, Colette Crutcher and Aileen Barr, was dedicated. The Lion Dancers performed, there were refreshments, the street was blocked off, the neighborhood was there, and Mayor Francesco Pignataro of Caltagirone, Italy, spoke eloquently. The famous Scala steps in his town were one source of inspiration for the 16th Ave. project. The citizens of this Italian town celebrate their stairway with an annual lighting of the stairs with hundreds of oil-filled cups called *coppi,* which create astounding patterns of light.

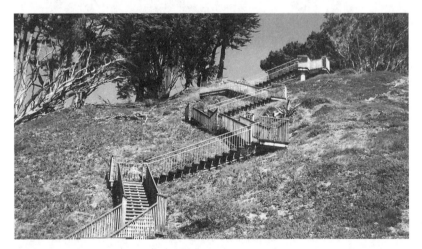

Grand View Park *Peter Nagy*

I could see the tiled steps from the bus just before we stopped. I was amazed how brilliant the colors were even under such bad weather conditions. The overall design with changing patterns and colors were most impressive. As we approached the last tiers, there were even some mirrors. I counted the steps in each tier and got a total of 162. With my altimeter watch, I measured the total height at 100 feet. —R. F., a walker from Southern California

⬛ As you reach the fifth landing of the Moraga Stairway, glance to the left. The Golden Gate Bridge and its two towers should be visible. You will be alerted to shifts in optical illusion during the walk.

⬛ At 15th Ave. turn right and walk to Noriega. Turn left and walk on the lower portion of Noriega. Turn right on 14th Ave. (near No. 1751), and bear left along the upper section of Ortega. The hill on the corner of Ortega and 14th Ave., also being restored by the California Native Plant Society, is a large expanse of exposed Franciscan Formation outcropping. No. 601 Ortega (1953) is built on it. The house is

Grand View Park Stairway   *Mary Burk*

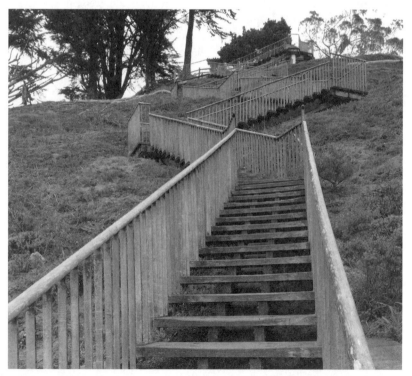

one of the most dramatically sited residences in San Francisco. Two other houses were subsequently built on neighboring lots, mitigating the drama of the entire hill.

◢ Turn right on Cascade Stairway, an unexpected tuck-in and right-of-way on the east side of No. 601. From the base, Twin Peaks is clearly in view. From the 50th step, the two towers of the Golden Gate Bridge coalesce into one.

◢ At the top of Cascade, the street signs read "Pacheco 900" and "Funston 1800." Follow Funston to the right, walking on the odd-numbered side for ocean views between the houses. Next to No. 1850 is a redwood house atop the hill; plantings adorn the wood stairway in front. The cascading garden of succulents is a source of delight for all who stop and look at it. Houses on the odd-numbered side date from the 1970s.

◢ At Aerial (opposite the stairway), turn left onto Pacheco. Turn right on Pacheco to the triangular piece of land at 12th Ave. The residents interested in gardening and keeping the neighborhood beautiful work diligently together on this project. Ascend the curved stairway to 12th Ave.

◢ Continue left on 12th Ave. to the intersection of Rockridge and Cragmont across from Golden Gate Heights Park. Cross Cragmont, and turn left to 12th Ave.

◢ At No. 2026 12th Ave., cross the street and follow the paved path into the park. Turn left at the playground, and continue right on the path to the roundabout and sitting area at the top. Follow the paved path to descend the hill. Turn left at the tennis courts, and continue to Rockridge. Cross Rockridge to Funston.

◢ Carl E. Larsen, a Danish restaurateur, loved this area. His chicken ranch on 17th Ave. and Noriega was the site for an annual Easter egg hunt for neighborhood children. By the time of his death in 1924 at age 84, he had given the city 6 acres of land in Golden Gate Heights, including Golden Gate Heights Park.

◢ Walk on Funston to Aerial Stairway, one of the longest in San Francisco. It is surrounded by cypress trees and ice plant. Descend Aerial Stairway to 14th Ave. at No. 1920. Turn right and continue on 14th Ave.

◢ Now in the 1800 block of 14th Ave., you walk past Ortega Way Stairway next to No. 1883. This is the other side of the hill facing Ortega. Just past the mature acacia, a profile view of the chert outcropping on the Ortega and 14th Ave. hill comes into view. No. 1843 faces the Franciscan rock outcrop. The rock always reminds Adah of Nathaniel Hawthorne's short story "The Great Stone Face." In it, a child, Ernest, spends many hours looking at a rock formation in New Hampshire's White Mountains with his mother. His favorite of her stories was the legend of "a child who should be born hereabouts who was destined to become the greatest and noblest personage of his time, and whose countenance in manhood should bear an exact resemblance to the Great Stone Face." Ernest is recognized as its likeness.

◢ Next to No. 1795 14th Ave., descend Mount Stairway, where you may notice that a neighbor has been gardening with native plants. The stairway ends across from No. 1801 15th Ave.

◢ Turn right. Continue on 15th Ave. past Noriega to the retaining wall. Ascend the stairway to upper 15th Ave.

◢ Cross upper 15th Ave. to the Grand View Stairway. Concrete piers support a wood stairway accented by a wood handrail, and a very nicely sited wood-slat bench on the landing allows you to look out west over the ocean. An information placard about Grand View Park is strategically placed at the bottom of the stairs.

◢ Ascend the stairway into Grand View Park, a superb place to watch the sunset. The 1.1-acre park is habitat for several native plant species: bush lupine, beach strawberry, bush monkeyflower, and coyote bush. The rare and endangered plants here are the Franciscan wallflower and the dune tansy. Restoration of Grand View Park is under the aegis of the Yerba Buena Chapter of the California Native Plant Society and the Natural Areas Division of the San Francisco Recreation and Parks Department. Both local neighbors and Eagle Scouts participate in volunteer work.

◢ You pass two landings with wood benches. At the second bench, take the first footpath to the left for a view of the city. Pass the mature Monterey cypress trees. Continue walking around to the right (the path narrows). Stop and look at the Golden Gate Bridge to observe an optical illusion. You can see what looks like three towers on the bridge, which change as you walk around the footpath. As you walk farther, in the distance, Golden Gate Park is a sea of green cutting a swath between the Sunset and Richmond neighborhoods.

◢ Look west, and you can see the VA Medical Center standing on the hill at the farthest point west; George Washington High School is the large building east of it. The curving street that snakes through the park is 19th Ave. With its two spires, St. Anne's Church is the Sunset neighborhood's most familiar peach-colored icon. Views to the west feature the Sunset Reservoir and demonstrate the relative flatness of the neighborhood stretching out toward the ocean.

⬦ You're walking on a hill of windblown sand, but underneath it is chert, layered at odd angles, reddish in color, and embedded with pieces of radiolarian, the one-cell marine rhizopod. Geologists have found radiolarian hundreds of feet below sea level and have dated samples at 140 million years. Walking near remnants exposed as the ocean receded, you feel connected to the beginnings of time.

Graffiti on the Moraga Funston Stairway   *Mary Burk*

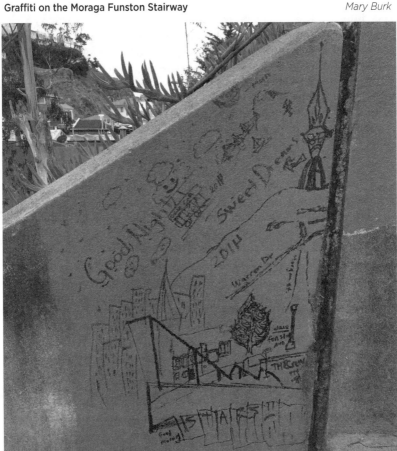

◢ Continue on the footpath to the stairway. Then turn to look and
see that a tower on the Golden Gate Bridge has almost disappeared.
Turn left to descend the wood stairway to 14th Ave. On the last landing, you have a panoramic view from Mt. Sutro to the Golden Gate
Bridge. At the bottom of the stairway, now only one tower on the
bridge is visible.

◢ Turn left on 14th Ave. Walk to the intersection of 14th Ave., 15th
Ave., and Aloha. Veer left on Aloha to Lomita. At the intersection of
Lomita and Aloha, there's a triangular section with a small stairway
enhanced by shrubs and flowers. Bear left, descend the stairway to
Lomita, and continue to 16th Ave. Veer left to your beginning.

Further Rambling

The Hidden Garden Steps project for the 16th Avenue Stairway between
Lawton and Kirkham was completed in December 2013. It is the second
tiled stairway created by the artists Colette Crutcher and Aileen Barr, who
also created the tiles for the Moraga Stairway. Crutcher and Barr have
been tapped to beautify another San Francisco stairway in 2014 in the
Bayview as well. Neighbors and other volunteers have given of their time
and money and have coordinated many cleanup efforts for the stairway
over the last three years in order to make this gorgeous stairway tiling
project a reality.

To enjoy this stairway, from the end of this walk, walk one more
block north to Lawton, and turn left to reach the 16th Avenue Hidden
Garden Steps on your right. Descend and then look back as you take each
flight down so that you can enjoy all the glazed, ceramic glory. Neighbor
and local business names adorn many of the tiles, which are floral and
bright.

If you wish to visit to Golden Gate Park, take MUNI Bus #66 Quintara to 9th Ave. and Judah (two blocks from the park). Points of interest
in the park include the San Francisco Botanical Garden, Conservatory
of Flowers, de Young Museum, the California Academy of Sciences, and
the Japanese Tea Garden. Irving is also one of the Inner Sunset's densest
shopping streets.

Links & Conundrums

St. Francis Wood

This neighborhood's streets and open spaces are not exactly circular. (*Circular* applies loosely because mathematicians only allow 360 degrees to a circle.) St. Francis Wood has, in some places, an irrational street design, as an architect friend once described it. A street in this neighborhood can even diverge into two segments that share the same name. To find your way without losing the rhythm of the walk, be sure to look for the numbers on the street signs, such as "San Pablo 300" and "Santa Paula 70."

Andrew S. Hallidie's cable car conquered the Clay St. Hill in 1878 and made Nob Hill accessible. But O'Shaughnessy's Twin Peaks Streetcar Tunnel conquered the hilly western district of Twin Peaks in 1918 and made it accessible. And this tunnel spelled the beginning of St. Francis Wood development. If you look at a topographic map of the area, you can see why it was so difficult to develop the western side of Twin Peaks—hills of chert (part of the Franciscan Formation) and high sand dunes. By implication, it is also an area of wind and fog. But there are views, fresh ocean air, and a forest of trees that Adolph Sutro planted after he bought 650 acres of the Rancho San Miguel land grant back in 1880. Sutro was one of very few historically important entrepreneurs who loved the western part of San Francisco and lived there (Carl Larsen was another). Others favored Nob Hill.

Another person who loved the west side of San Francisco was Duncan McDuffie. He was an environmentalist, president of the Sierra Club (1928–1931 and 1943–1946), and believer in the principles of the City Beautiful movement that was gaining momentum throughout the country in the early 1900s. He also was a partner in the Mason & McDuffie real estate company. McDuffie enjoyed the western section of San Francisco, and the company was interested in purchasing land here. The only amenity missing was good transportation.

Michael O'Shaughnessy, chief engineer at the time, proposed building the Twin Peaks Streetcar Tunnel to solve this city problem. Finally, in 1912, construction began. Real estate developers began to buy land. Mason & McDuffie bought 175 acres of the Rancho San Miguel from the four Sutro heirs who were free to sell after their father's will was declared null and void. Mason & McDuffie planned to develop St. Francis Wood. The company had previously developed several neighborhoods in Berkeley, Crescent Park, Claremont Upland, and Park Hills that expressed the idea of open space, trees, shrubs, and parks as important ingredients in designing a city neighborhood that is pleasing and nourishing for human beings.

Henry Gutterson, the chief architect hired by Mason McDuffie to plan out St. Francis Wood in the same spirit as Daniel Burnham's City Beautiful plan, with circular streets, spaces between houses, wide sidewalks, parks, open space, and lots of trees, helped realize this vision in the

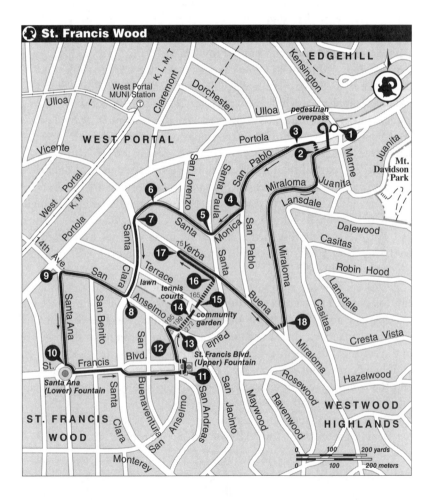

QUICK-STEP INSTRUCTIONS

1. At Portola, take pedestrian overpass from Kensington to Miraloma. Right on Miraloma.

2. Before No. 2 Miraloma, descend stairway to Portola and left to San Pablo.

3. Left on San Pablo to Santa Monica.

4. Cross the street, and walk right onto Santa Monica to Santa Paula.

5. Continue right on Santa Monica. (Check the street signs carefully.)

6. Pass San Lorenzo and follow curve to the left on Santa Monica to Santa Clara.

7. Left on Santa Clara to San Anselmo.

8. Right on San Anselmo to Santa Ana.

9. Sharp left on Santa Ana to St. Francis Blvd. and the Santa Ana Fountain (or Lower Fountain) and roundabout.

10. Left on St. Francis Blvd. Pass San Benito and San Buenaventura to San Anselmo and the St. Francis Blvd. Fountain (or Upper Fountain) and plaza.

11. Ascend the stairway to the right. Walk toward the left. Descend stairway on your left. Right to street sign that reads "Santa Paula End" and San Anselmo 200."

12. Walk on San Anselmo past the white fire hydrant No. 6 and trees. Cross San Anselmo to No. 195, and continue right to No. 199.

13. Immediately after No. 199, turn left to descend Terrace Walk Stairway.

14. Right to walk around the community herbal garden to 165 Terrace Dr.

15. Ascend the continuation of Terrace Walk Stairway. At the end of Terrace Walk, you are directly across from street sign "Yerba Buena 100."

16. Left on Yerba Buena to Nos. 75, 44, and 34.

17. Retrace your steps to the "Yerba Buena 100" street sign, and continue past Santa Paula and San Pablo. Just past Maywood, ascend stairway on the left to Miraloma.

18. Left on Miraloma to your beginning.

neighborhood of St. Francis Wood. The company hired the finest landscape designers, the Frederick Law Olmsted Jr. Office of Boston, and the architects like Gutterson, who graduated from the University of California, Berkeley, and the École des Beaux-Arts in Paris.

During World War I, Mason & McDuffie's business was marginal. (In 1915, for instance, the company's total income amounted to $5,000.) However, Gutterson persisted with his vision of nature and city living, and eventually Mason & McDuffie received loans from friendly banks.

Developers financed Gutterson's vision for St. Francis Wood, and the city of San Francisco received a jewel of a neighborhood. After the first street-car ran through the West Portal Tunnel in 1918, the business of selling St. Francis Wood houses increased substantially. By 1925, more than 400 families were living in the development.

WALK FACTS

Artistic planned living based on the Beaux Arts school of Paris in this neighborhood is tranquil and yet on a grand scale. Nearby neighborhoods wish they were as elegant.

Other neighborhoods grew up around St. Francis Wood after it was designed. Parkside was developed in the 1940s and 1950s, and San Francisco State University moved to its new campus in 1953, which was carved out of the Parkmerced neighborhood.

Shopping is nearby, at the Stonestown shopping mall and at the Ocean Avenue shopping thoroughfare near Junipero Serra and Sloat Boulevard.

Bus Routes & Parking

PUBLIC TRANSPORTATION: MUNI Bus #43 Masonic and #48 Quintara. Farther away, several Metro lines stop at West Portal Station. For Muni bus or Metro information, call 311 (outside San Francisco, call 415-701-2311).

PARKING: You can park on Ulloa at Kensington with no restrictions on time. There is also street parking available, usually allowed for up to two hours. But also look for street-cleaning times posted in the neighborhood to avoid getting ticketed or towed.

WALK 12 DESCRIPTION

There are several entrances into St. Francis Wood. You enter through one of the back doors so that you can end close to the beginning of the walk. There are two alternatives. For a most unusual beginning, you can start on the north side of Portola Drive at the border of the Edgehill neighborhood on Ulloa and Kensington, where there are no parking restrictions except for street cleaning. Walk across the Portola pedestrian overpass to Miraloma and Marne on the south side of Portola. The second alternative is to come by bus and begin at the pedestrian overpass at Miraloma near Marne.

◢ If you elect the first alternative, you will see an aged Monterey pine whose multiple trunks and cascading branches provide a canopy for the overpass. The West of Twin Peaks district is a forest of subneighborhoods: West Portal, Monterey Heights, Mt. Davidson, Sherwood Forest, and others. In spite of this and the hilly terrain, lot sizes are spacious, and vegetation augments the sensation of space. Look across Ulloa toward the Edgehill neighborhood, a beautiful scene.

◢ Make a right turn on Miraloma toward No. 2. It is a very large house with a tiled roof and fits in comfortably with the corner. Look around and you will see the tip of the cross on Mt. Davidson. Descend the short stairway on the right to Portola. The traffic noise on Portola is a reminder to listen and compare noise levels as you walk throughout the city. At the bottom of the stairway, you come to an unusual sight. The New Zealand Christmas tree (*Metrosideros excelsa*) at the base of the stairway has red aerial roots that travel down the trunk of the host tree until they touch ground. At that time, they start to develop into a separate trunk, much like a banyan tree. This only occurs in areas where there is optimum fog and dampness. Another area in the city where you will find an example of this is at the entrance of the San Francisco Botanical Garden, opposite the Japanese Tea Garden and adjacent to Stow Lake.

◢ As you walk left on Portola, you will see a sign that reads "Positively no trespassing" at the bottom of a discontinued, derelict stairway. Next to it is No. 1135, beautifully terraced with rocks. A standard with a light on top is next to the garage. The street sign here reads "Portola 1200, San Pablo 000." Walk to San Pablo following the curve. Pass another entrance that has a concrete standard inscribed with the name "St. Francis Wood." On the hilly part of the left sidewalk on which you are walking, there are unusual mounds of English ivy. The red flowering gum tree (*Eucalyptus ficifolia*) is the street tree here. They are abloom with orange blossoms usually in August and September. The house roofs range from deeply sloped to extending to the hip of the house. The sidewalk has little insets of brick squares. There is abundant foliage, an inviting entrance to the neighborhood.

Traveler, there is no path. Paths are made by walking.
　　　　　　　　　　　　　　　　　　　—Antonio Machado y Ruiz

⊿ You cross the street onto Santa Monica where the street sign reads "Santa Monica End." Continue to Santa Paula. At the intersection, at No. 101 Santa Monica, is a house of many gables. How many do you count? Test yourself to see if you can count the same number three times in a row.

⊿ Continue to the right on Santa Monica where the house numbers are below 100. The direction of the curving streets is confusing, so check the signs carefully. Pass No. 94 on the left, and take a look at No. 90 (the number is on the side of the house). This English-style house, built of natural concrete in 1921, has a low, wavy wood roof and mullion windows. It was designed by Henry Gutterson. The present occupants are only the second owners of the home. When they moved in, they had the roof reshingled. They asked the roofers to save the moss, which they then donated to the collection of the Strybing Arboretum (officially known as the San Francisco Botanical Garden at Strybing Arboretum).

⊿ Across the street, No. 85 Santa Monica is another Gutterson English-style stone house, built from Idaho sandstone in 1925, a true classic and favorite in St. Francis Wood. The house is angled, and next to it

Santa Ana Fountain   *Mary Burk*

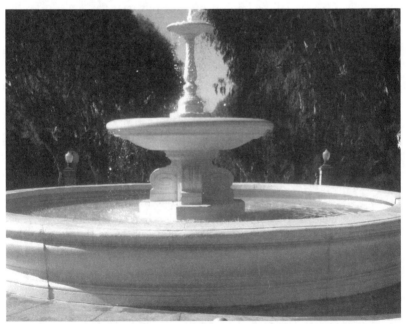

is a large hydrangea plant. A St. Francis sculpture is niched near the front door. The landscaping around the house is tastefully constructed with a variety of shapes of foliage and a variety of trees, the oldest of which dates back to the 1890s, when Sutro planted them.

◢ At the intersection of San Lorenzo on the left, the street sign states "Santa Monica 50." In the center of the street, there is an open space with benches. New trees have been planted, and some old, enormous Monterey pines are established here. At the V-shaped part of this rounded triangle, there are two street signs—"Santa Monica 33–55" and "Santa Monica 30." Walk on Santa Monica 30. A short, but useful stairway was built at No. 30 Santa Monica with six slabs of concrete that lead into the backyard.

◢ At the corner of Santa Monica and Santa Clara No. 40, turn left. Cross the street at the sign that reads "Yerba Buena 000," and walk on the right side of Santa Clara past Terrace. The St. Francis Wood Home Association office blends imperceptibly into its environment at No. 101 Santa Clara. A park and playground surround the structure in the back. All homeowners are members of the association that manages community property—parks, gardens, tennis courts, gateways, and the Children's Common in the public areas.

◢ Continue walking on Santa Clara to San Anselmo. Turn right on San Anselmo to walk to Santa Ana. London plane trees line the length of San Anselmo. Originally the developers wanted each circle block to have the same street trees and the same style houses, but the plan was not entirely successful. At Santa Ana, make a sharp left. The trees along the street here are ficus. Hebe was planted near the curve. Santa Ana is one of the flat streets and was one of the first developments in St. Francis Wood. The canopy of vegetation is sparse because many of the trees have only recently been planted. Compared to other streets, it seems almost bare.

◢ You are now at Santa Ana No. 100 and St. Francis Blvd. No. 300, the location of the Santa Ana Fountain (the residents call it the Lower Fountain) and roundabout. It was designed by supervising architect John Galen Howard, dean of the School of Architecture at the University of California, Berkeley from 1903 to 1924. He also designed the pillar entrances and sidewalk patterns. Short stairways are at every corner of the roundabout. Turn left at the fountain onto St. Francis Blvd. The light standard reads, "The Circle." Continue left on

St. Francis Blvd., and walk past the corner of San Benito No. 100 and St. Francis Blvd. No. 400.

◢ Continue on St. Francis Blvd. The traffic on the boulevard is heavy. There are stop signs on some of the corners, but watch and be aware. Use the crosswalks. The trees in the St. Francis Wood neighborhood are impressive in their number, sizes, ages, and variety, especially the eucalyptus on St. Francis Blvd. From a distance the lines of trees seem to continue forever, and in a sense, they will. Some of the trees were brought in from the 1915 Panama-Pacific International Exposition.

◢ The houses on the boulevard are formal and stately. No. 405 St. Francis Blvd. dates to 1948. You are now at St. Francis Blvd. No. 500 and Santa Clara No. 300. Cross Santa Clara, and continue on St. Francis Blvd. A large oval median is the introduction to the ornamented St. Francis Blvd. Fountain (or Upper Fountain as the residents call it) designed by Gutterson in 1912. A mature magnolia flourishes at No. 531. You can see the brush cherry trees near the corner of San Buenaventura where they line the street near No. 50. No. 600 St. Francis Blvd. is a stucco house, with curved living room windows extending almost down to grass level. Baroque decoration surrounds the front door. No. 630 St. Francis Blvd. is built in the Southwest architectural style with overhangs to shade it from the sun.

◢ You arrive at the St. Francis Blvd. Fountain at San Anselmo. There are stone benches on each side of the boulevard for you to take your time to enjoy the long view of the fountain within its setting. St. Francis Blvd. is the main axis and the imposing main entrance of the neighborhood with streets radiating from it. Walk across San Anselmo to the plaza area. All around the walkway by the plaza are red brick squares inscribed with the names of donors who contributed to the 1998 restoration of the plaza's sculptured features, like the fountain. On the left side of the wall is a plaque with a portrait of Duncan McDuffie and a tribute to his vision for St. Francis Wood.

◢ Ascend the stairway on your right near San Andreas. Walk left past the fountain and plaza area, and descend the stairway to the left. Turn right to the intersection where the street sign reads "Santa Paula End" and "San Anselmo 200." Continue walking on San Anselmo, past the white fire hydrant No. 6 and the stand of a dozen London plane trees. This is where the fun begins!

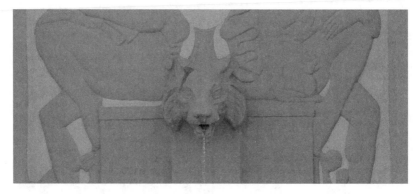

Detail of large fountain *Mary Burk*

◢ Cross San Anselmo, and turn right to No. 195. Walk past No. 199, and immediately turn left to the entrance of Terrace Walk Stairway, which begins with a gravel-lined pathway with shrubbery all around. (Incidentally, if you walk beyond No. 199 San Anselmo, you are then on Santa Paula.)

◢ The stairway is well situated here in terms of the rhythm and length of the walk. Descend this stairway of redwood steps, which feels more pliant to the feet than other types of wood. The landings are concrete and the railings are metal. Assorted foliage grows around the sides. The stairway descends to No. 266 Terrace Drive. A community herbal garden is on the right, a tool shed is in the center, and tennis courts are on the left.

◢ The Terrace Walk Stairway continues on the left side of No. 165 Terrace Drive. Ascend the stairway onto a pathway to the street. You will be directly across from a street sign that reads "Yerba Buena 100." Turn left to No. 75 Yerba Buena, a house designed by Julia Morgan and built on a rise. A curved brick stairway leads up to the front door framed with Corinthian columns. The house has a more formal appearance than other houses on the block. The windows are wall length.

◢ Walk to No. 44 to see the delicate filigree gate. A eucalyptus tree with an impressive and unusual gall-like swelling is in front of No. 34. The growth appears to have been caused by a cellular division that went out of control—somewhat analogous to cancer but not as serious. The leaves from the eucalyptus trees on this block were formerly picked by the San Francisco Zoo to feed the koala bears. At the present time, the horticulture staff collects branches daily from various areas of the

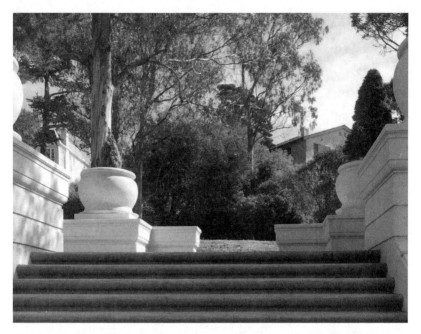

Detail of stairs up to large fountain   *Mary Burk*

city, including McLaren Park, Visitacion Valley, Stern Grove, Candlestick Park, and Monterey Blvd. The koalas are finicky eaters and are offered at least five different varieties of eucalyptus daily.

◢ Return to Santa Paula, and continue walking on Yerba Buena. Pass San Pablo on your left, and continue on Yerba Buena toward Miraloma. No. 136 Yerba Buena has a very attractive stone chimney. Looking at it may remind you of sitting around a cheery fireplace and making s'mores at summer camp as a child. Continue on Yerba Buena past Maywood. Ascend the stairway on the left at the "Miraloma End" sign. Continue walking left on Miraloma to your beginning.

Further Rambling

If you wish to link St. Francis Wood with Mt. Davidson (Walk 13), walk to Marne and Miraloma. Proceed with directions for Walk 13. Another graceful link can be made with Edgehill (Walk 14). Walk across the pedestrian overpass at Portola and Miraloma to Kensington. Turn right on Ulloa, and proceed with directions for Walk 14.

Now You See It, Now You Don't:
Discover the Fog & Light of San Francisco

Mount Davidson

At 938 feet, Mt. Davidson is the highest hill in San Francisco. Known in the 1850s as Blue Mountain, it was renamed Mt. Davidson in 1911 to honor George Davidson (1825–1911), first surveyor of the mountain, internationally renowned scientist, and president of the California Academy of Sciences. Mt. Davidson became a city park in December 1929.

The Mt. Davidson neighborhoods are part of the enormous residential area west of Twin Peaks, which is surrounded by subneighborhood sections: Sherwood Forest (there's a Robin Hood Drive here), Westwood Highlands, and Miraloma Park. Larger homes can be found west and north of Mt. Davidson; the smaller ones are in the eastern Miraloma section. Feel free to ramble through the various surrounding neighborhoods. You will see magnificent views beside Miraloma School at Omar and Myra, and from Marietta Drive and Bella Vista.

The idea of a cross on Mt. Davidson originated with James Decatur, and an Easter service was first held there in 1923. At that time there was a 40-foot wood cross, which was replaced three times over the years. Finally, in 1934, the present 100-foot stone cross was erected with a time capsule and the original deed to Mt. Davidson placed in the base. One week before Easter of that year, President Franklin Roosevelt lit the cross via telegraph. The city annually illuminated it during Christmas and Easter seasons, and thousands of people attended the Easter Sunday sunrise services on the mountain.

However, in 1996, the US Appeals Court ruled that the religious symbol violated the constitutional separation of church and state. In 1997, San Francisco approved the sale of the cross and surrounding one-third acre to the Armenian American Organization of Northern California for $26,000. It is preserved as a historic landmark in memory of the 1.5 million Armenian victims of genocide perpetrated by the Turkish government from 1915 to 1918.

Walking the trails that cut across slopes covered with pine and euca-lyptus can be confusing because the Department of Recreation and Parks has not yet put up signage. Adah's challenge was finding the trail leading to the desired exit. Though she tried the walk at different times with vari-ous friends, the problem continued. An engineer friend finally solved it by advising, "Keep it simple." It worked. Adah found two beautiful stone stairways, a breathtaking view, trails with blackberries (edible) and Coast strawberries (inedible), ferns, and wildflowers, including forget-me-nots, nasturtiums, and monkeyflowers. Breathing ocean air and eucalyptus, you will know that you are in the city but also feel quite removed from it.

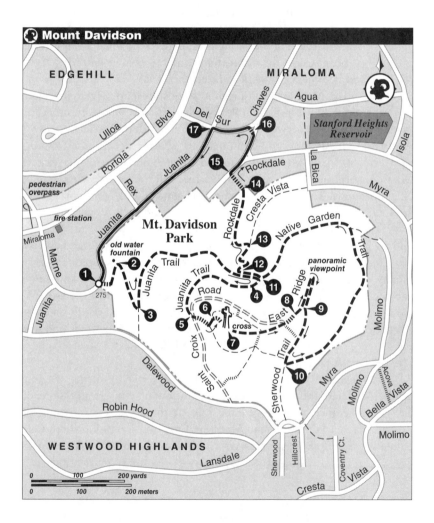

QUICK-STEP INSTRUCTIONS

1. Begin on Juanita at No. 275. Ascend the stone stairway beside the house.

2. Left on Juanita Trail. Right at the nonfunctioning drinking fountain.

3. Turn left and ascend the trail. Where Cresta Vista Trail joins your route on the left by the tall sequoia tree, continue up toward the right.

4. At junction (ahead) with Native Garden Trail, switchback right, staying on the Juanita Trail.

5. Cross the access (St. Croix) road, and ascend a stone stairway and then a log stairway bearing left.

6. Right and ascend a log stairway to the back of the cross on the summit.

7. Walk to front of the cross toward the cliff side.

8. Left and descend wood stairway. Follow the East Ridge Trail to the panoramic overlook.

9. Retrace your steps to the first left. Descend south on a medium-steep gravel and log road, the Sherwood Trail.

10. After the fifth log, bear left on the Native Garden Trail, which descends and partly circumnavigates the peak. Ascend a tree root stairway.

11. Where the Native Garden Trail joins the Juanita Trail at the switchback, turn right to descend.

12. Right at the first path, Cresta Vista Trail, across from the tall sequoia tree. It switchbacks a couple times before reaching the junction with the Rockdale Trail.

13. Left at junction onto Rockdale Trail. Path narrows just before the stairway.

14. Descend stone stairway to Rockdale St.

15. Right on Rockdale St.

16. Left on Chaves. Descend corner stairway to Del Sur. Left on Del Sur to Juanita.

17. Left on Juanita to your beginning.

Two other entrances to the park are the St. Croix Trail at No. 39 Dalewood and the Sherwood Trail at the #36 Teresita MUNI bus stop on Dalewood. The St. Croix Trail has two stone stairways ascending to the summit. (Another stone stairway is closed at this time.) An upper stone stairway is near Juanita Trail. Beyond this stairway on St. Croix Trail to the summit is a large rock outcropping with hanging greenery. The Sherwood Trail meets the East Ridge and Native Garden Trails.

To traverse Mt. Davidson and exit by another trailhead, from the summit follow the East Ridge Trail to the panoramic lookout, and partly retrace your steps to descend along the first left-branching road, the Sherwood Trail. Keep going ahead where the Native Garden Trail branches left. You can descend the Sherwood Trail down to Myra and Dalewood, where you can take MUNI Bus #36 Teresita to Forest Hill Station or the Balboa Park BART station.

You could also walk left on Myra around the park on the city streets to La Bica. Turn right on La Bica, walk one block to Rockdale, turn left for a block, and then continue, as described above, to your beginning at No. 275 Juanita.

While historic trail names were still being assigned throughout the Bay Area in 1935, when the Works Progress Administration blazed the trails on Mt. Davidson, they did so without signage. We have settled on two nonhistoric names to help out the adventurous reader-walker. The Sherwood Trail is named for the street at the end of the trail. The Native Garden Trail was always a footpath and not included in the original park.

WALK FACTS

George Davidson originally named this geographical center of San Francisco Blue Mountain for the blue lupines he found growing wild on the hillsides.

The movie *Dirty Harry* used Mount Davidson as a location for a ransom scene that took part in front of the trail up to the cross. The scene where Dirty Harry gets his man was dramatically shot from directly below the cross.

Easter sunrise services have been held on top of Mount Davidson since 1923, and the view from the top at sunrise is heavenly every day of the year.

Bus Routes & Parking

PUBLIC TRANSPORTATION: MUNI Bus #43 Masonic and #48 Quintara. Farther away, several Metro lines stop at West Portal Station. For MUNI bus or Metro information, call 311 (outside San Francisco, call 415-701-2311).

PARKING: There is street parking, which is usually allowed for two hours, but also look for street-cleaning times posted in the neighborhood to avoid getting ticketed or towed.

NOTE: Portions of the trails are narrow and rocky. Watch your step. The park is under reconstruction. Information here is the latest available.

WALK 13 DESCRIPTION

⊿ Begin west of Mt. Davidson, at the stone stairway next to No. 275 Juanita. Your route is upward. Blackberries growing along the stairway taste delicious when in season. When you reach a nonfunctioning drinking fountain (still useful as a landmark), ascend toward the right. At the next fork, climb toward the left. Wildflowers grow alongside the trail. Where the Cresta Vista Trail joins your route on the left, near the tall sequoia tree, ascend to the right. Where the Native Garden Trail joins your trail at the point of a switchback, turn sharply right to continue up the Juanita Trail to St. Croix Road.

⊿ Cross St. Croix Road (for vehicles). Ascend the stone stairway, turn left, and continue on the log stairway. Turn right, and ascend the tree root and log stairway behind the cross to the summit. At the summit, walk to the front of the cross toward the cliff side, where you will see views of the East Bay hills and the Campanile (Sather Tower) at the University of California, Berkeley.

⊿ Turn left and descend the wood stairway. Follow the East Ridge Trail to the panoramic viewpoint. Retrace your steps, but bear left before the wood stairway. Descend and continue along a medium-steep gravel and log path, the Sherwood Trail.

⊿ Soon after the fifth log where the Sherwood Trail meets the Native Garden Trail, turn left. The trail descends and partly circumnavigates the peak, overlooking the Miraloma Park neighborhood. You will pass two tall wire fences and ascend a tree root stairway. Watch your step. The barren path leads to the wooded area that eventually rejoins the Juanita Trail.

⊿ At the junction, turn right to descend Juanita Trail. Almost immediately you reach the junction of Cresta Vista Trail. Look for the tall sequoia tree. Turn right down the Cresta Vista Trail. It gently veers left and right a couple times before reaching the junction with the Rockdale Trail.

Jamaicans don't say, "Goodbye." They say, "Walk good."

⊿ Turn left onto Rockdale Trail. At Rockdale, cross over a log you'll see buried in the path. It has a yellow reflector attached to it. Continue on the path to a stone stairway that ends on Rockdale St. Turn right

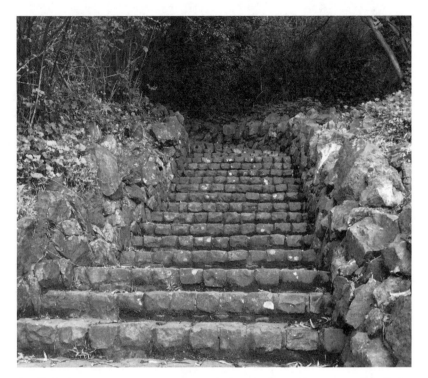

Juanita Stairway   *Mary Burk*

on Rockdale. Veer left on Chaves, and descend the corner stairway to Del Sur. Turn left to Juanita and your beginning.

◢ On the way, you pass Franciscan Formation outcrops at the park's edge and some seeps (active in winter) that support ferns, eucalyptus, and other lush vegetation.

Further Rambling

If you wish to link Mt. Davidson with Edgehill (Walk 14), walk across the overhead pedestrian skyway at Portola and Miraloma to Kensington. Turn right on Ulloa, and proceed with directions for Walk 14.

◢ Another graceful link can be made with St. Francis Wood (Walk 12) by walking to Marne and Miraloma; proceed with the directions for Walk 12.

Chert, Hideaway Paths, & Open Space

Edgehill

The Edgehill houses perched 600 feet above sea level allow their occupants to see extraordinary sunsets, glistening Pacific Ocean waters, and 32 miles to the northwest, the Farallon Islands, which are part of the sovereignty of San Francisco. In return for these favors of nature, the residents have accepted narrow roads and troublesome curves, as well as periodic landslides. The San Francisco Fire Department has learned to send up extra lengths of hose and not to send up the hook-and-ladder truck. Delivery companies likewise do not send up large trucks. Developers have learned to expect noisy opposition from residents to their plans for building more homes on precarious land. Still, a few developments have been built on the precipices. And problems have arisen.

The most recent major one occurred in 1997 when residents noticed cracks in the road that increased in size the next day. Under the direction of consulting engineers and geologists Cotton, Shires & Associates, Inc., crews worked vigorously to stabilize Edgehill Way and prevent more damage to homes at both the top edge and the bottom of the cliff. Several residents were forced to vacate their homes. The story will unfold as you walk, beginning at the base of the circle, from bottom to top, from the newest addition to the oldest.

The instability and fragility of the houses on this walk have fascinated Adah for years. People you may meet along this walk may share their personal accounts of their encounters with you as you foray through the neighborhood. Although Adah's diary-style accounts of meeting local residents and of how the area has changed the last few years are still very fresh, as the past has shown, the rocks on this mountain may choose new edits through the very nature of their instability, and new slides may force us to redesign the walk for future safety.

WALK FACTS

Edgehill is part of the San Miguel hills, which run southwest from Twin Peaks to Mount Davidson, Hawk Hill, and Edgehill.

Raptors like red-tailed hawks, black hawks, caracaras, and even an albino turkey vulture have been seen along the ridge that Edgehill belongs to. Keep your eyes peeled, and bring binoculars.

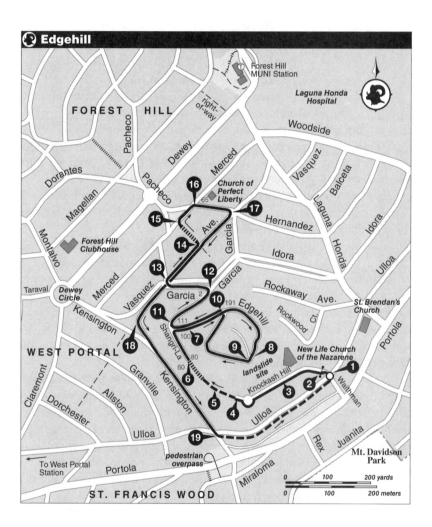

QUICK-STEP INSTRUCTIONS

1. Begin at Ulloa and Waithman.

2. Enter resident gate of Knockash neighborhood. Walk on the left side of the street.

3. Walk past New Life Church of the Nazarene on the right and Knockash Hill residences on the left.

4. Bear right at "Edgehill Mountain Open Space" sign onto path.

5. From the top proceed downhill a few feet, and follow the upper path (stairway) to your right.

6. The open space area ends at No. 60 on unmarked Shangri-La Way. Continue to the end of Shangri-La Way to No. 100 Edgehill Way, and turn right.

7. Continue up Edgehill Way, and follow the one-way sign around the mountain.

8. Pass No. 280, and continue past the mailboxes, Nos. 300 and 350 Edgehill, and the driveway to the right, which is private property and, therefore, closed to the public.

9. Continue past fire hydrant labeled No. 8, and walk through wooded area.

10. Left at No. 191 Edgehill Way, and backtrack to No. 111 Edgehill Way.

11. Right at No. 111 Edgehill Way to No. 2 Upper Garcia.

12. Left on Upper Garcia to Vasquez.

13. Right on Vasquez to Pacheco.

14. Left on Pacheco, and descend stairway to Merced.

15. Right on Merced to Hernandez.

16. Right on Hernandez to Vasquez.

17. Right on Vasquez to Kensington.

18. Sharp left on Kensington to Ulloa.

19. Left on Ulloa to your beginning.

Bus Routes & Parking

PUBLIC TRANSPORTATION: MUNI Bus #43 Masonic and #48 Quintara. Farther away, several Metro lines stop at the Forest Hill MUNI Station. For MUNI bus or Metro information, call 311 (outside San Francisco, call 415-701-2311).

PARKING: Unlimited parking is available on Ulloa at Kensington.

WALK 14 DESCRIPTION

◢ Begin at Ulloa and Waithman, the entrance to Knockash Hill Rd., and walk through the pedestrian gate. This development of 13 homes, also known as the Knockash neighborhood, has undergone a metamorphosis since Adah began exploring the area in the 1980s. First, it was just a parking lot, and the church was the only structure here. But before that, it was the site of a stone quarry. After the horrific rockslide in January 1997, Adah felt she should wait until geologic conditions became more stable before including an Edgehill walk. In 2005, she revisited the area to scout, alone, with friends, and with people interested in seeing the neighborhood. Knockash Hill Rd. was a dramatic surprise. Since the area had changed so much since the 1997 landslide, Adah felt it was time to include it and that there was no choice but to begin the walk at Ulloa and Waithman. The area has remained stable since 2005, and the walk remains. And so we begin.

◢ Adah recalls her first reaction was: "How beautiful!" On the right, within 20 feet of the beginning, is a wall of layered red chert, built up over the last 100 million years. Her second reaction was: "Where did all these houses come from?" What a contrast in age between the 100-million-year-old wall and this new human-made walkway and brick border on the left—all within 20 feet of each other.

◢ Adah's research also included talking with residents and reading in the main San Francisco Public Library. The quarry work in the early 20th century had intensified the fragility of the steep cliffs, resulting in small rockfalls. The cliffs were not successfully stabilized until after the 1997 landslide. Wire mesh that covers the slope as you walk through Knockash is clearly visible. Although it may be difficult to visualize how it was done, according to records, 99 multistrand, double-corrosion-protected tieback anchors were used, and almost 1,200 linear feet of belt structures went into the design used in the hillside stabilization plan.

◢ The gray specks in chert are radiolarian, an aquatic plankton. Chert, one of the elements of the Franciscan Formation, was pushed up from deep water by volcanic upheavals. (You can see good examples of it from Mount Olympus to Diamond Heights and in the parking lot at the Randall Museum near Corona Heights.) Succulents grow on the hillside, and lichens abound on the rocks. A bit farther on, you see chert formations along both sides of the street.

- Pillars on the left and right sides of the road announce the New Life Church of the Nazarene. The congregation here is relatively small (church headquarters are in Kansas City, Missouri). The church celebrated its 100th anniversary in 2005. The hillside is terraced, and a small area is allocated for church parking.

- At the cul-de-sac end of Knockash Hill Rd. are two basketball hoops. (Young couples with children comprise the majority of homeowners in the Knockash subdivision.) Continue up toward the right on a narrowing path. There are two pillars and a sign that reads, "Edgehill Mountain Open Space, San Francisco Recreation and Parks Department."

- Knockash Hill Rd. is one of the entrances into the park. A descending dirt path introduces you to a wooded area. The path leads to corner pie-shaped steps behind a sitting area. Bear right on the upper path to walk on the rustic stairway that wends among the trees and leads to the residential area.

- A bench, a bit off the path, is an invitation to those who would like to sit and contemplate the serene setting of blue gum eucalyptus and Monterey pine and cypress and the height and steepness of the slopes.

Knockash Hill *Mary Burk*

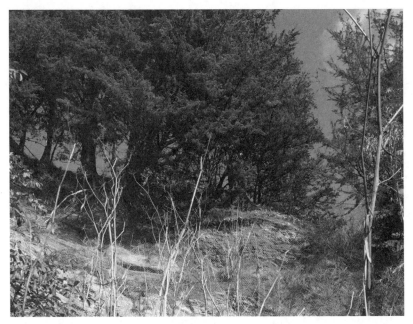

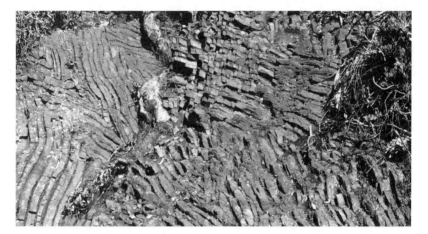

Detail of sedimentary rock on Edgehill   *Mary Burk*

Every month, dedicated volunteers plant native plants and grass, a successful venture; they also rid the area of invasive plants like ivy and ehrharta grass, which looks a little like green barley. Blue, yellow, and white flags mark sites of new plantings. Walk up log steps where wild onions sprout on the side of the stairs.

◢ As you come to the edge of the open space, you are now on Shangri-La Way. Its existence invites a great trivia question: What is the shortest "street" in the city that, although without signage, has a legal name known to residents but not to outsiders? The answer is Shangri-La Way. It extends from No. 60 to the metal horse at No. 100, a distance of only a few feet. The rest of Edgehill has one name—Edgehill Way. Shangri-La is the second entrance into the open-space park.

◢ No. 60 Shangri-La Way at the top of the hill, on your left, is built on steel stilts. No. 80 (on the right side) has an unusually long window wall. The owners of No. 56 enjoy a compelling view to the north, complemented by a patio. A bit farther on is No. 54 with an unusual exterior of concrete embedded with pebbles.

◢ No. 100 Edgehill at Shangri-La is unusual because of the two sculptures at the corner. You first pass a totem pole fabricated by a member of a Native American tribe in Washington State; the metal bear comes from Mexico. Now you are on Edgehill Way.

◢ As you turn right, you come across No. 111, one of the largest homes on the hill. No. 140 on the right side has beautiful stone steps. The stones that are an integral part of the architecture of many homes here come from the quarry. Across the street, on the other side of No. 121, you can see the canyon below. It is wild with trees, vines, nasturtium, wild onion, and some California poppies. No. 191 is at the end where the road around the mountain begins. No. 200 has a particularly appealing stone wall. No. 220, in the early days, was a speakeasy. No. 250 was the first house built on the hill in 1927 by the current resident's father. It incorporates, so pleasingly, huge boulders on the property (even embedding a mailbox into one) and redwood trees.

⊿ On walks through the neighborhood, Adah and I have both met neighbors out for their daily walks. And sometimes, the walking neighbors became a walking group. Several residents have lived in Edgehill for close to 50 years. They love living on the mountain.

Edgehill neighborhood was one of my husband's favorite areas in San Francisco. We lived there for 46 years. We saw the Farallon Islands on a clear day. We could see Golden Gate Bridge, the two tunnels beyond, and Forest Hills with its colorful houses and tile roofs that reminded us of the hill towns of Italy. We did have a lot of fog, but even then, it was very beautiful. The sunsets were magnificent. Sometimes they were orange, sometimes pink—there isn't a more beautiful place in San Francisco on a nice day.
—Former resident J. M.

⊿ The area between Nos. 275 and 301 is the site of the 1997 mudslide that destroyed part of the street and where a small modern house with solar heating was formerly located. After the slide, it was declared unsafe for occupancy, taken down, and destroyed. The retaining wall and additional metal fencing were erected as part of the stabilizing plan.

⊿ From No. 280, continue past the private driveway with mailboxes for Nos. 300 and 350 and the white fire hydrant with the number 8 printed on it. Continue walking into the wooded area of Edgehill Way.

⊿ Adah refers to this neighborhood as one of the most magical unblocks in San Francisco—a *rus in urbe*, or country in the city, if one can ever use the term. In Edgehill, you are suddenly transported. The paths are narrow, only one car wide, and the road is confined by a deep ravine on the left and the wall of chert on the right. Above, trees, eucalyptus and pine, hang down randomly. You may feel you are treading lightly on soft, easy earth. But it's not true. You are walking on crushed stone, formed like a macadam road from the 1800s. On the right side of the road, you can see layers of brick that were previously used on nearby property. (San Francisco accepted Edgehill gravel roads from the developer only as a public road to be driven on, but the city did not accept responsibility for its maintenance.)

- At No. 345 we're back in the city. Turn left at No. 191. At No. 111 Edgehill, veer to your right, and continue walking downhill to Garcia. Continue left on Garcia to Vasquez.

- Turn right at No. 150 to descend the little Pacheco Stairway, a series of steps and landings. The widest steps are at the base of Merced, where benches are built into the wall. As you descend, you might recognize how this stairway echoes the longer Pacheco Stairway in front of you and welcomes you to the adjoining Forest Hill neighborhood (for more, see Walk 15).

- Turn right on Merced, and continue until you come to Hernandez. The Church of Perfect Liberty at No. 65 Merced occupies a large white structure at the corner, a former residence. It has been in San Francisco since 1960 and has a congregation of 250 to 300 persons. Perfect Liberty is a religious group founded in Japan in 1924 by Tokuharu Miki, who died in 1938. The church's mission is to bring about world peace by living the precepts of "Life is art" and "Man's life is a succession of self-expressions."

- Continue right on Hernandez, and then turn right on Vasquez to Kensington. Turn left onto Ulloa, and return to your beginning.

Further Rambling

The end of this walk leads you directly into Walk 15, Forest Hill. A short respite in West Portal to the south a couple blocks, where shopping, restaurants, and specialty stores offer their wares, might be a welcome break between these two lovely walks. Stern Grove with 63 acres to explore is also nearby, or visit on a Sunday in summer for free concerts. Walk 13 for Mount Davidson is also nearby; from Ulloa, walk south to cross Portola, turn left on Rex, and continue to Juanita. But this recommendation is only for the heartiest of walkers.

Marienbad in San Francisco

Forest Hill

It's not the longest stairway in the city or the steepest; it's not the most charming, nor the most personal. Filbert and Vallejo Stairways, Oakhurst Stairway, Vulcan and Harry Stairways, and Pemberton Stairway, respectively, have these attributes. However, the grand Pacheco Stairway is by far the most elegant in all of San Francisco. An urn of flowers 20 feet in diameter introduces this long stairway placed amid forest and lawns. The stairs themselves are 18 feet wide with balustrades, columns, and patterns of stones repeating into the distance; as Adah says, they lend a dreamlike, rococo quality to the setting. Think of Alain Resnais's film *Last Year at Marienbad*; how easily the Pacheco Stairway could fit into the surroundings of Marienbad. This luxurious walk of curves and curlicues reiterates the innate elegance of this stairway and its sylvan setting.

Forest Hill was originally part of the 4,000-acre Rancho San Miguel, granted in 1843 to José de Jesus Noe, the last Mexican alcalde (mayor) of San Francisco. After California became part of the United States, the 11 ranchos that comprised the town were subdivided. In 1880 Adolph Sutro bought 1,100 acres of Noe's rancho; the Crocker Estate bought the rest.

Public transportation became easily accessible to the western part of the city after the Twin Peaks Tunnel was built. In anticipation of this development, the Newell-Murdoch Company began subdividing the Forest Hill tract in 1912, cutting down much of what had been extremely dense forest planted by Adolph Sutro and his Arbor Day volunteers. Difficult engineering and construction problems were solved in a most aesthetic manner by Mark Daniels, the landscape engineer (and former general superintendent of the US National Park Service), who deserves a plaque commending his design of curving streets that follow terrain contours, generous stairways, ornamental urns, concrete benches, balustrades, parks, and terraces. Daniels also designed the grand staircase at Dewey and Pacheco, up to Magellan.

The fine city planning Daniel Burnham intended for all of San Francisco was carried out in Forest Hill. This City Beautiful planning follows

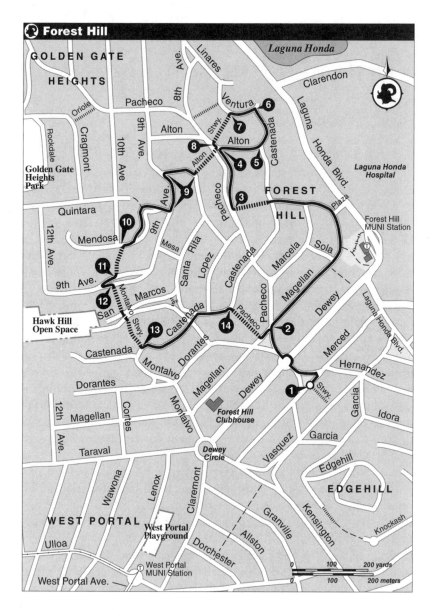

the axis of Pacheco, north into Forest Hill, and south into the Edgehill neighborhood—if only the 1906 earthquake hadn't interrupted the 1905 plan, alas.

Forest Hill also has the distinction of having the largest concentration of Bernard Maybeck homes in the city. Maybeck is Adah's favorite California architect of the early 1900s who espoused the Craftsman style

QUICK-STEP INSTRUCTIONS

1. Begin at Merced and Pacheco. Cross Dewey Boulevard carefully to Pacheco and Dewey, then walk north on Pacheco to Magellan.

2. Right on Magellan, and continue past Sola and Marcela to the stairway next to No. 140 Castenada. Ascend to No. 334 Pacheco.

3. Right on Pacheco to Alton.

4. Right on Alton to Castenada.

5. Left on Castenada to Ventura.

6. Left on Ventura to No. 60 Ventura.

7. Ascend stairway to Pacheco, No. 400.

8. Cross the street to crosswalk at Pacheco and Alton street sign. Walk up 10 steps to upper Pacheco, and cross the street to No. 399 Pacheco. Continue ascending Alton Stairway.

9. At the top of stairway, next to No. 60 Sotelo, bear right, then turn left on 9th Ave., and then right on Mendosa.

10. Descend the Montalvo Stairway between Nos. 91 and 99 Mendosa.

11. Curve right around planted median, and then turn left to lower 9th Ave., next to No. 2238 9th Ave.

12. Descend Montalvo Stairway on lower 9th Ave. past San Marcos to Castenada.

13. Left on Castenada to grand Pacheco Stairway next to No. 249 Castenada.

14. Descend to Pacheco and Merced and your beginning.

of architecture. He used redwood for the exteriors, brought light into the interiors, and related living areas to gardens. Maybeck taught in the School of Architecture at the University of California, Berkeley. He died in 1957 at the age of 95.

No. 266 Pacheco was the first house built in Forest Hill (1913). In 1918, the year the first streetcar went through the Twin Peaks Tunnel, the Forest Hill Association was organized. They set home-building standards, such as a minimum 1,500-square-foot interior and 19-foot setback from the sidewalk. They taxed themselves to maintain the grounds, and because the delightful, nonconforming streets and stairways did not meet city specifications, the association was also responsible for them. After years of controversy and court action, the city, in 1978, accepted responsibility for streets and curbs in Forest Hill, but the residents remain responsible for stairways and sidewalks. The association is still an active community group, which meets regularly at the Forest Hill Clubhouse.

WALK FACTS

Major renovations of the Forest Hill Clubhouse, at No. 381 Magellan, were completed in 2013. The building is one of the best examples of Maybeck's work. It is both Adah's and my favorite on this walk.

On Sunday evenings, perhaps after a nice walk, take in a donation-only music concert at the Forest Hill Christian Church, home to Forest Hill Concerts. Concerts start at 6:30 p.m., and the church is at 250 Laguna Honda Blvd.; call 415-890-4342 to see who's playing.

Bus Routes & Parking

PUBLIC TRANSPORTATION: MUNI Metro L, M, or K to Forest Hill Station; #43 Masonic; #44 O'Shaughnessy. For MUNI bus or Metro information, call 311 (outside San Francisco, call 415-701-2311).

PARKING: There is metered street parking available; metered parking is usually available for up to an hour, and free street parking usually allowed for up to two hours. But also look for street-cleaning times posted in the neighborhood to avoid getting ticketed or towed.

WALK 15 DESCRIPTION

⬦ Begin the walk at Merced and Pacheco (technically known as Forest Hill Extension, because these homes were added later) to experience the gradual change of view—distant to close-up—of the lovely Pacheco Stairway. The beautiful entrance to the Forest Hill neighborhood is echoed here by the short Pacheco Stairway (Walk 14), with its long, curving concrete benches flanked by griffins and a large, ornamental urn in the center green.

⬦ Proceed into Forest Hill on Pacheco to reach Dewey. Walk north on Pacheco to Magellan; turn right and walk on the right side of Magellan. The trees and the uniform height of the homes provide a counterpoint for the variety in the exterior walls, the shapes and materials of the roofs, and the symmetry, coherence, overall appeal, and mellowness of the block. No. 255 Magellan is a slate-roofed, brick house with gardens on three lots, surrounded by a wrought iron fence with gilded finial darts.

◢ Next to No. 201 Magellan is a right-of-way that goes to Dewey. Beyond Sola you soon pass the back of the Forest Hill MUNI Station. After Plaza you continue to the end of Magellan. Turn left on Castenada to ascend the stairway next to No. 140, a Maybeck-designed house of 1924. The carved grapevines along the eaves (representing fecundity) blend in so well with the surrounding vegetation that you almost fail to see them. At the top of the stairs, you're at No. 334 Pacheco. Turn right.

◢ At Alton, turn right and then left on Castenada to Ventura. The best weather pattern in Forest Hills is in this northeast section.

◢ No. 2 Castenada has a magnificent, award-winning cactus garden of many varieties (in addition to more recent plantings), which complements the Southwest style of the house. The owner continues to augment his collection with other varieties of plants.

◢ Turn left on Ventura, and ascend the stairway next to No. 60, which continues up to No. 400 Pacheco and No. 70 Alton. A retired resident we met informed us that he takes great delight in gardening; we found marigolds, liatris, red hot pokers, pincushions, honeybush, and even some vines. The area sparkles with color.

◢ You are at the change-of-name point in the block. Alton begins at No. 70 and continues to the east. From No. 400 the street becomes Pacheco and runs northwest of the Alton Stairway. How is a person to know of these vagaries without getting lost a few times?

Pat F. has what, in her Southern family, is known as a "bump of direction," that is, a natural, perfect sense of direction.

◢ Walk a few feet to the crosswalk to cross the street safely at the Pacheco and Alton street sign. Ascend the 10 steps to upper Pacheco, then cross the street to No. 399 Pacheco, and continue ascending the Alton Stairway.

◢ At the top of the Alton Stairway, you are next to No. 60 Sotelo. To the left, at No. 51, is a 1914 Maybeck house with an off-center, octagonal, pulpitlike balcony; the sides are decorated with redwood shingles and an open carved-wood design. You are surrounded by craftsmanship and subtle design that blends into the natural environment.

◢ Bear right on Sotelo, and then turn left on 9th Ave. to go right on Mendosa. Descend the Montalvo Stairway between Nos. 91 and 99 to upper 9th Ave. Turn right to follow the curve around the planted

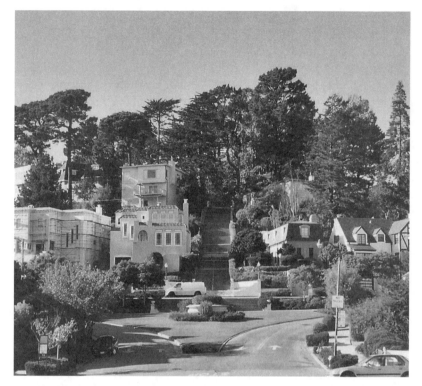

Pacheco Stairway from Dewey Blvd.   *Peter Nagy*

median, and arrive at lower 9th Ave. It's a small price to pay for the aesthetic experience of walking on divided streets.

- Descend the Montalvo Stairway on lower 9th Ave. (next to No. 2238), past No. 199 San Marcos. You pass a backyard with formal hedges and cobblestone walls and arches. Turn left at Castenada. No. 270, at the corner of Lopez, is another Maybeck home. Built in 1918, it is a three-story, shingled residence with bays and dormers.

- Next to No. 249 Castenada is the Pacheco Stairway. As you descend the grand Pacheco Stairway to the street, thoughts of Jerry Healy, the first superintendent gardener of this elegant tract neighborhood (he was also known as the "Mayor of Forest Hill") may come to mind. Healy planted geraniums and marguerites so that the area was a mass of red and white. The neighborhood association still uses splashes of bright colors in their plantings like Healy did, and the *byzantina* (lamb's ear), *Salvia,* and viola pansies planted in recent years have been lovely.

◢ If you would like to see the Maybeck-designed Forest Hill Clubhouse at No. 381 Magellan, turn right at the bottom of the stairway. Otherwise, descend to Dewey Blvd. and then Merced, to your beginning.

Further Rambling

To link Forest Hill with Edgehill (Walk 14), from Merced, turn left and follow the Edgehill route Steps 16–19. Then follow Edgehill route Steps 1–14 to return to your beginning at Dewey and Merced.

Grading & Sliding, Fog & Drip

Forest Knolls

The rock formations in San Francisco, built up through millions of years of sediment pressure and tectonic upheavals, appear to grade and slide in a geological pattern we can only guess is discernible in thousand-year intervals. The rock around San Francisco quietly informs us of its past through its presence. The rocks are red and crumbly—sometimes they are made up of granite pushed up from South America, and sometimes it has become serpentine, or sandstone. All of these rock types make up the slopes of Mount Sutro, one geologic chunk at a time.

Forests are good at holding onto fog. And because the western section of San Francisco receives significant fog, when it settles into treetops like you find in Forest Knolls, you suddenly have a kind of rain forest. After Adolph Sutro planted thousands of eucalyptus, Monterey pines, and cypresses (here and on Twin Peaks) to hold the soil, the land became better established. Sutro followed Nebraska's example in the 1870s to help establish Arbor Day in California and, during his term as mayor of San Francisco, had schoolchildren help plant trees.

Many of the eucalyptus trees planted in Sutro's time have been cut down or have fallen down. Because they have a shallow root system, their life span is a mere century—very brief for a tree. Yet the abundant trees in Forest Knolls still provide habitat and food for many birds, including larger birds like hawks and owls. Trees also provide subtle screening between houses, so look closely to see edifices on stilts or to spy the birds and ocean. And, of course, pay close attention so that you do not miss any of the elusive stairways.

The Forest Knolls neighborhood is bounded by 7th Ave. in the Sunset neighborhood on the west, and by Clarendon and the Twin Peaks neighborhood to the east. Situated on the south slopes of Mt. Sutro (918 feet), it was largely developed for housing in the 1960s. Though the architecture is similar throughout the curving streets, the area is rich in geologic history. Over a period of about 10,000 years, alluvial deposits and layers of sand have blown in from the beach. The terrain can be unstable in times of earthquakes and heavy rains.

After a landslide occurred in 1966, a 10-year building moratorium was declared for the area. Beneath layers of sand, Mt. Sutro is composed mostly of red chert, the dominant rock in the Mt. Davidson and Twin Peaks area. It accounts for the high elevations in this part of the city. Chert is one of the hardest components of the Franciscan Formation—it is little affected by wind and rain, yet it can erode into unstable clay. Homes built in the 1980s have required expensive engineering to strengthen them against landslide and earthquake damage.

Residents with whom Adah talked over the years expressed delight in living in a forest, a nonurban section of the city because a few blocks away they can board MUNI to catch a movie, visit the library, or go to the store. And although Forest Knolls receives a disproportionate amount of fog, not once did anyone we meet mention it; in a slight wind, the wisps of the fog that linger merely make the area seem more mysteriously charming. As you walk along here, you'll enjoy breathing in the fresh ocean air.

WALK FACTS

Forest Knolls was Adolph Sutro's hunting preserve and part of the one-twelfth of San Francisco he owned.

Forest Knolls stairways are all known as lanes.

The Mount Sutro Urban Forest is very close by and has trails, mostly without signage, that offer enjoyable walks through the woods in sun or fog. These two forests present contrasting natural respites from the city around them.

The West Portal Shopping area and the MUNI West Portal Station are both nearby, offering shops and restaurants along a tree-lined boulevard.

Bus Routes & Parking

PUBLIC TRANSPORTATION: MUNI Bus #36 Teresita. Farther away, several Metro lines stop at Forest Hill Station. For MUNI bus or metro information, call 311 (outside San Francisco, call 415-701-2311).

PARKING: There is metered street parking available; metered parking is usually for up to an hour, and free street parking is usually allowed for up to two hours. But also look for street-cleaning times posted in the neighborhood to avoid getting ticketed or towed.

WALK 16 DESCRIPTION

◢ An unusual stairway presents itself to us as a starting point. It's Ashwood Lane Stairway, 0.2 mile from the Oak Park and Forest Knolls beginning, and it illustrates two principles: It provides a valuable shortcut into the Forest Knolls neighborhood from an important thoroughfare, Clarendon, and the stairway path has the atmosphere of the mountain area that Adolph Sutro enjoyed so much. If you do not wish to use this alternate beginning, start your walk at Oak Park and Forest Knolls.

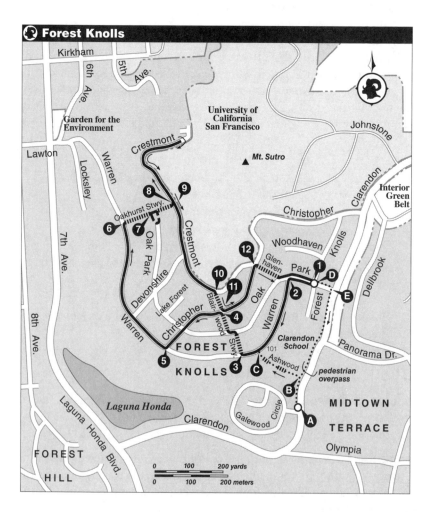

QUICK-STEP INSTRUCTIONS

A. *Alternate beginning:* Begin at the "Galewood Circle Dr." street sign on the west side of Clarendon.

B. Walk into Ashwood Lane, to the right of Galewood Circle Dr.

C. Continue on the stairway until No. 101 Warren. (Continue with No. 2 below.)

1. Begin at Oak Park and Forest Knolls.

2. Bear left on Warren.

3. Ascend Blairwood Lane Stairway to Christopher.

4. Bear left on Christopher to Warren.

5. Right on Warren to Oakhurst Stairway (to the left of No. 398 Warren).

6. Ascend Oakhurst Stairway.

7. Right into cul-de-sac of Oak Park, and then return to Oakhurst. Right on Oakhurst to Crestmont.

8. Detour left on Crestmont, then return to Oakhurst.

9. Continue on Crestmont to Blairwood Stairway.

10. Descend Blairwood Stairway to Christopher.

11. Left on Christopher to Glenhaven.

12. Descend Glenhaven Stairway to Oak Park and your beginning.

D. *Alternate ending:* Continue to Clarendon.

E. Right on Clarendon to your beginning.

◢ Continue the walk at Oak Park and Forest Knolls, just off Clarendon. Turn left on Warren. Across from No. 113 Warren is the Blairwood Lane Stairway, which you ascend to Oak Park. Foliose lichen is encrusted on the railings. Lichens flourish where there are no competitive plants and where the air is clean. Vertical gardening is practiced here because of the terrain. It's delightful to see the success of this ornamental vegetation endeavor. Sedum has been planted on the left among the other vegetation.

◢ At Oak Park (next to No. 301), cross the street, and find a continuation of Blairwood Lane Stairway a few feet to the left. Walk up to Christopher (next to No. 301). The plantings across the street are beautifully terraced with pines, eucalyptus, ice plants, century plants, and marguerites. To the right you can often see fog hanging in the eucalyptus trees on Mt. Sutro.

In 1995 two footprints were found in a sandy shore of what was once a steep sand dune, now hardened to gray sandstone, along Langebaan Lagoon near Cape Town, South Africa. Discovered by David Roberts, a South African geologist from the Council of Geoscience, they have been identified as the oldest fossilized tracks of an anatomically modern human found to date. They measure about a woman's size-seven shoe and have been dated back 117,000 years.

◢ Turn left on Christopher. On the slope to the left is a multitrunked pine covered with lichen. Continue to Warren, and turn right. The attractive single-family dwellings, pastel-colored and angled, were designed thoughtfully to allow for maximum light, both reflected and direct.

◢ Across from No. 399, you ascend what must be considered a "floating stairway," the Oakhurst Stairway, hidden among the eucalyptus. (The -*hurst* so often attached to English village names means "wood.") The hillside on the left has been leveled, and drains have been installed. The slope is a sea of emerald green grass in winter. You're in a landscape of eucalyptus, bottlebrush, daisies, weeds, ice plants, and mallow. And the Pacific Ocean extends as far as the eye can see.

◢ The climb is steep. Halfway up the zigzag stairway, you might sit on the steps to admire an extraordinary wide-angle view as, perhaps, an ocean liner glides east.

◢ Finally at Oak Park, you turn right into a narrow walkway that leads into the cul-de-sac. A series of single-family dwellings have been built on your left. Nos. 560 and 550 were built in 1980, the others in 1990 and 1991. I-beams have been driven deep into the rock to provide safety for these homes in this landslide area.

◢ Return to the stairs, and continue your ascent to Crestmont. Orange lichen on the green handrails and blue *Vinca major,* among the variegated greens of ferns, ivy, and eucalyptus, create visual interest near the long retaining wall ahead, which delineates Sutro Woods (Adolph Sutro's former hunting grounds) and the edge of the urban forest.

◢ Turn left and explore this part of the Forest Knolls neighborhood a bit before proceeding right. Each house on Crestmont has a garden reached via stairs. Between Nos. 95 and 101, near the white fire hydrant, is the Blairwood Lane Stairway. Descend the stairway down to Christopher, and turn left. Just ahead now you can see the Glenhaven Lane Stairway, well-lit in the evenings for winter strolls. Descend down Glenhaven Lane Stairway to Oak Park Drive. On Oak

Park, next to No. 191, you can see hillside chert, a sediment outcropping ranging from beige to red, as if the mountain was peeking out next to the stairs.

◢ Now walking down Oak Park, you see a monkey puzzle tree in the distance. Soon you arrive at your abbreviated beginning. Or alternatively, continue east on Oak Park Drive to Clarendon (the alternate beginning) at the entrance, so to speak, of the Forest Knolls neighborhood.

Further Rambling

For those walkers who would like to experience the Ashwood Lane walkway and stairway, begin at the west side of Clarendon, just south of the pillars of the pedestrian overpass at the sign for Galewood Circle, a mini-neighborhood. Begin the walk at A, and then continue with B, C, and Step 2. Working an overpass into the walk feels rather exciting, and this alternative lets you feel a little closer to the neighborhood as a local.

Take Clarendon, an important corridor street, to the Twin Peaks, Forest Hill, or Golden Gate Heights area. Food is available in the Irving and Judah sections of the Sunset and the Market and Castro sections of Upper Market. At Lawton and 7th Ave. in the Sunset District, you can explore the Garden for the Environment, a demonstration and teaching site sponsored by the Haight-Ashbury Neighborhood Council.

Oakhurst Stairway   *Peter Nagy*

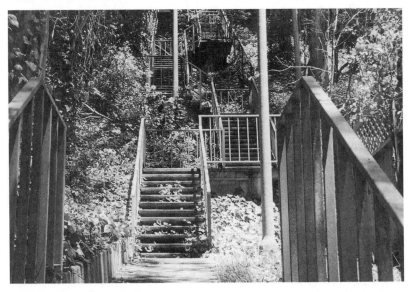

Angle vs. Contour

Twin Peaks Foothills

In the middle of the city is an outcropping of rock, predominantly composed of chert, basalt, shale, and sandstone. Subdividing the area was a daunting task, but short streets and an interconnecting network of stairways resolved the problem. While the short streets are in many ways comparable to those on the eastern side of the city, these hills are higher than either Telegraph Hill or Russian Hill. The Upper Market, Eureka Valley, or Castro (all names in use) neighborhood is also known for its gardens, cooperative neighbors, and attractive, renovated Victorians.

Like Adah, I also enjoy tracking changes in city neighborhoods we've both been exploring over the years. In 1981, Adah wrote of that wonderful feeling of luxury she felt the first time she descended the wide, upper section of Pemberton. "It was one of the most graceful stairways in the city." The heavy rains of 1982–83, however, precipitated the deterioration of the older brick stairs and the crumbling of the sandstone wall entrance along Clayton. To prevent the stairway and the wall from collapsing, the Department of Public Works (DPW) installed 4-foot-square beams. Work dragged on.

A decade later, the residents and DPW began to work cooperatively on the project. In the year 2000, the defective and dangerous stairs were redesigned according to City code: fabricated with concrete, but terra-cotta in color and stamped with a brick-shaped mold. New landscaping was also planted: Japanese maples at the landing and shade-tolerant ground covers of *Vinca major* and jasmine, plus colorful annuals. The last portion to be finished, the wall along Clayton, was replaced with an attractive terra-cotta concrete wall 20 years later (better late than never), and the new improvements should last longer too.

Public Works engineers, landscape architects, and others involved in the Pemberton project enjoyed the challenge of designing a stairway that met code requirements for safety, as well as the aesthetic requirements of the community. The teamwork between the city department and the neighbors began with patient and thorough neighborhood grassroots planning, spearheaded by a Pemberton resident. In 2002, former resident Rodney Ruskin presented a drinking fountain in memory of his wife, Myra, and her contributions to the community. The fountain is situated on the Villa Terrace landing.

WALK FACTS

The Twin Peaks Foothills are more commonly referred to as Upper Market, Eureka Valley, or the Castro District. Some boundaries and divisions by street and signage are debatable. However, on this walk, you stay above the Castro and Eureka areas but can consider yourself very Upper Market.

A very old road that started out as a road for farmers living in the outside lands (the southwest part of San Francisco) to bring products to market, Corbett used to extend southwest much farther. Part of it was later renamed Junipero Serra. In the mid-1800s, it was a toll road leading to the Ingleside and Ocean House Racetracks.

Bus Routes & Parking

PUBLIC TRANSPORTATION: MUNI Bus #37 Corbett. For MUNI bus information, call 311 (outside San Francisco, call 415-701-2311).

PARKING: There is metered street parking available; metered parking is usually available for up to an hour, and free street parking is usually allowed for up to two hours. But also look for street-cleaning times posted in the neighborhood to avoid getting ticketed or towed.

WALK 17 DESCRIPTION

◢ Begin at Romain and Corbett. Cross Corbett and turn right. As you pass the No. 660 mailbox, you will see a surprise public stairway; however, it leads to a private driveway. Therefore, continue on Corbett, and turn left on Graystone and then right onto Copper Alley Stairway. Descend to Corbett.

◢ Turn left and continue on Corbett. The odd-numbered side of the street offers views. Next to No. 555 Corbett is a framed view of downtown San Francisco. Rooftop Middle School (the Nancy Yoshihara Mayeda Campus) for children in grades five through eight is to the left at No. 500. A rock mosaic covers a small portion of the outside wall with the name "Rooftop School." The wall inside the playground features a large mural. Continue past Iron Alley Stairway at No. 495 Corbett, happily rebuilt and reopened after a long-needed restoration.

Walk to the intersection of Clayton. For your safety, use the crosswalks to enter the Neighborhood Garden at the tip of Clayton and Corbett, across the street from the Pemberton Stairway. It is one of the best-designed scraps of land we have. Professional gardeners consider

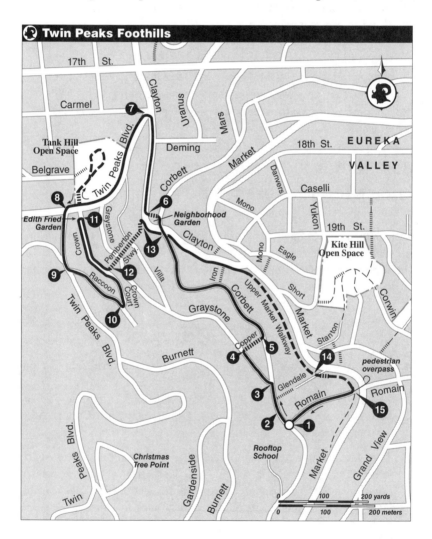

Twin Peaks Foothills

QUICK-STEP INSTRUCTIONS

1. Begin at Romain and Corbett.
2. Cross Corbett and turn right. Continue to Graystone.
3. Left on Graystone.
4. Right on Copper Alley Stairway. Descend to Corbett.
5. Left on Corbett, past Iron Alley, to Clayton intersection. Cross at crosswalks to corner Neighborhood Garden. Ascend stairway to Clayton.
6. Right on Clayton to Twin Peaks Blvd.
7. Left on Twin Peaks Blvd.
8. Cross Twin Peaks Blvd. and walk up stairway to see the view from Tank Hill. Walk around hill and back, descending same stairway, to the boulevard. Turn right to the crosswalk. Turn left and cross the boulevard.
9. Continue on Twin Peaks Blvd., past Mountain Springs, to Raccoon Dr.
10. Bear left on Raccoon Drive to Crown Ct. Sharp left at the bottom of the hill. Walk past No. 127 Crown Ct., and continue on asphalt and stone path to Crown Terrace.
11. Continue toward end of Crown Terrace. Return to 130 Pemberton Place and 98 Crown Terrace across from Pemberton Stairway.
12. Descend stairway to Clayton.
13. Right on Clayton. Walk on right side to Market. Continue right onto Upper Market Walkway.
14. Descend and cross Glendale. Ascend stairway to continue on Upper Market Walkway to Romain.
15. Right on Romain to your beginning.

it a gem, and urban explorers are delighted to discover it. In this small space, there is much to keep you alert—so many levels and grades to explore and a variety of materials to be sensitive to. Scattered throughout the garden are jade, several varieties of *Salvia, Clematis,* black-eyed Susans, both yellow-and-brown and orange irises, and a Norfolk Island pine.

The impact of the Neighborhood Garden is greater than that of the immediate neighborhood. Over the years, Adah has seen people in their cars stop, roll down the windows, and thank whoever is working there for the beauty of the garden. The garden has been a volunteer effort since 1960. After the death of Drew Siegal, who first transformed the area into a garden, friends have continued to maintain and refine it. Many people now volunteer their time to maintain it. To prevent soil loss on the slope during the rainy season, Christopher J. Smith used stones from the Sierra Nevada configured in aesthetic patterns. Although he never thought his degree in theater design would be applied to his new interest in garden design, he has used brick, stone, and concrete judiciously. Signage near the park asks visitors to respect neighbors, visit quietly, and to not enter certain planting areas, but this garden is open and welcoming to all.

◢ Ascend the stairway to Clayton. Turn right on Clayton, and continue to Twin Peaks Blvd. Turn left onto the boulevard, and walk on the right sidewalk. Pass Crown Terrace, and ascend the short stairway to Tank Hill, one of the last bastions of native wildflowers the city possesses. Again, the interest of one person who has consistently worked to weed and plant on Tank Hill has enriched our lives and has encouraged others to help more and more. Walk upon the covered reservoir, installed in 1894 by the Spring Valley Water Company, and enjoy an unobstructed view of the city—take in Lands End to the west, Hunters Point to the south, and downtown San Francisco to the east. Look again.

If we cross the road, taking care not to be cut down by some rash driver—for they drive at a great pace down these wide streets— we shall find ourselves on top of the hill and beneath shall see the whole of London lying below us. It is a view of perpetual fascination at all hours and in all seasons.
—Virginia Woolf, *The London Scene*

◢ Descend the same stairway and turn right. At the pedestrian crosswalk, turn left to cross the boulevard to another beautiful spot where the association named for it contributes to the maintenance of the Edith Fried Garden. A bench adds another friendly aspect to this small triangle of land in the neighborhood.

◢ Continue south on Twin Peaks Blvd., past Mountain Springs, then on to Raccoon Drive, and bear left. Raccoon offers a spectacular view, unusual for an access road. Continue down to Crown Court, but mind the road as it is open to vehicles. A few homes are sited on the right. Take a sharp left, and walk past No. 127 Crown to No. 125 where the view across the Bay looks like a landscape portrait of the sunny East Bay and Mount Diablo State Park northeast of Danville, about 30 miles away. The stone house on your left (No. 110) is well located in the cul-de-sac. Crown Terrace is part of the district that was known as Little Italy in the 1930s. The Bank of Italy, which subsequently became

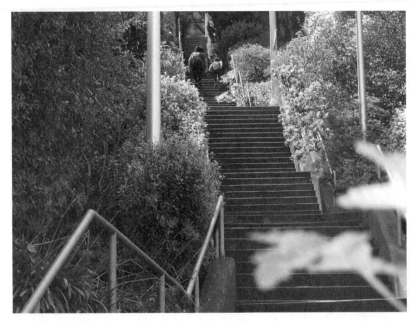

Pemberton Stairway   *Annette Hovie*

Bank of America, held many of the mortgages on these homes (many of which were foreclosed on during the Great Depression).

- Continue to the end of Crown Terrace, then return to the intersection signed "130 Pemberton Place/98 Crown Terrace" to descend Pemberton Stairway. Continue past Graystone Terrace and Villa Terrace to Clayton.

- Turn right on Clayton and walk on the right side to Market. The street sign at the corner reads "Clayton End & Market 3350." Veer right onto the Upper Market Walkway that descends to street level. Cross Glendale and ascend the short stairway back to Upper Market Walkway.

- Continue to Romain, and turn right to your beginning.

Further Rambling

If you would like to walk some other little-known short streets and stairways in the area, cross Market St. at the light, and head north toward Short, Eagle, and Yukon Streets. You can also combine this tour with Walk 18 (Upper Market) or Walk 20 (Eureka Valley), depending on whether you'd like to head north or south. Both directions are equally enjoyable.

Narrow Streets, Privacy & Quiet Among the Planets

Upper Market

If at any time over the last century, you had walked from Ocean Beach at the western end of the city and finally arrived at 17th St. and Clayton (where this walk begins), and you did this once roads were built so you weren't traversing vast dunes, or crossing dairyland, or brush, you still would have really worked up to it, vertically speaking. The land begins sloping up the eastern side of 19th Ave. at about 4th Ave. and Parnassus, where the University of California, San Francisco Medical Center is located, and the rise to here is most noticeably higher than the ocean shoreline behind you. At 17th St. and Clayton, you are even higher again, entering a relatively unknown area where cut-off streets may confuse you, there is no shopping, and city walkers relish the opportunities presented in this hilly area for excellent urban exploring. A 40-year resident of Upper Terrace says that when people realize how difficult it is to maneuver cars along the narrow streets, they usually drive away, leaving behind the privacy and quiet.

WALK FACTS

This walk sits just above the Castro Street neighborhood and Cole Valley.

Natural springs from the Joost Mountain Springs Water Company made the land below Twin Peaks muddy and valuable.

Once the Twin Peaks Tunnel project started in 1914, the spring that Behrend Joost utilized was destroyed, and his feud over water with the Graystone family ended in failure for both of them.

Bus Routes & Parking

PUBLIC TRANSPORTATION: MUNI Bus #37 Corbett. For MUNI bus and Metro information, call 311 (outside San Francisco, call 415-701-2311).

PARKING: There is metered street parking available; metered parking is usually available for up to an hour, and free street parking is usually allowed for up to two hours. But also look for street-cleaning times posted in the neighborhood to avoid getting ticketed or towed.

WALK 18 DESCRIPTION

◢ Begin at the intersection of 17th St. and Clayton under the green "17th Street 4600" sign. Walk down 17th St. about 50 feet just past the Monument Way Stairway. You can see how the apartment complex is sited on the Franciscan Formation outcrop. Return to ascend the stairway, an abrupt, ambitious beginning, though the rise only extends from 449 to 476 feet. At the top of the stairway, you can enjoy an open view of Sutro Forest and the neighborhoods around it, as well as the Marin Headlands, Point Reyes, the Golden Gate Bridge, and Mt. Tamalpais. You're now on Upper Terrace, where multiple dwellings dominate the street.

◢ Turn left on Upper Terrace, and walk to the right of the large, circular, raised-concrete planting area in the middle of the street. In 1887 Adolph Sutro placed the Mt. Olympus monument *The Triumph of Light,* a sculpture of a Greek goddess, here to denote the geographical center of San Francisco. If you ascend the stairs, you'll see that the pedestal is still present, but the sculpture has been removed. The 360-degree panorama of the city is partially concealed by trees; walk up the monument steps for a look.

I love to annotate the phenomena of the city. I can be as solitary in a city street as ever Thoreau was in Walden.
                              —Christopher Morley, "Sauntering"

◢ Next to No. 480, descend to No. 227 Upper Terrace (lower section). Turn left. Both the quality of the light and the small distinctive houses contribute to an attractive ambiance. Continue on Upper Terrace to Clifford Terrace. Turn right. At the bottom of the slope, walk down six steps, cross Roosevelt Way to No. 475, and descend the Roosevelt Way Stairway.

◢ Turn left on Lower Terrace to Levant. At the corner, you see Corona Heights (see Walk 19) to the northeast.

◢ Turn left on Levant and, a few feet away, right onto Vulcan Stairway. A local resident says he knows every step intimately—he used to walk up all 218 steps daily. It is a miniature Shangri-La, even though the stairway plantings are overgrown. Neighbors have traditionally worked together to beautify the gardens and walks. On one side of the stairs is a row of remodeled, eclectic, mostly turn-of-the-century cottages. Well-designed patios and decks extend living outdoors, and skylights open interiors to natural light. English ivy covers the slopes, and in different seasons you can also find fuchsia, rhododendron, azaleas, and hydrangeas in bloom. Residents of the hill to whom Adah and I have both spoken love living here.

◢ At the bottom of Vulcan Stairway at Ord, turn right and walk to Saturn Stairway. An area with embedded red bricks on the left and a terraced area with high stone walls to the right visually leads you to

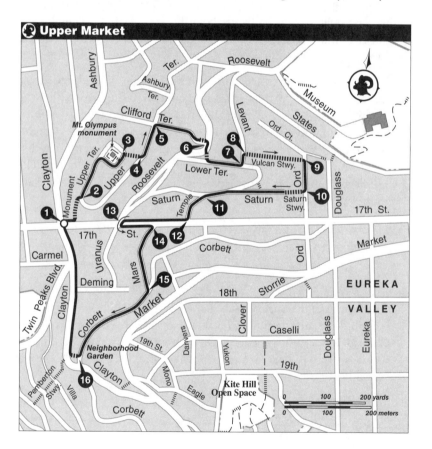

QUICK-STEP INSTRUCTIONS

1. Begin at 17th St. and Clayton. Ascend Monument Way Stairway to Upper Terrace.

2. Bear left and then right around Mt. Olympus monument.

3. Next to No. 480 Upper Terrace, descend stairway to No. 227 Upper Terrace.

4. Left on Upper Terrace.

5. Right on Clifford Terrace, descend six steps, and cross Roosevelt Way. Next to No. 475 descend stairway to Lower Terrace.

6. Left on Lower Terrace.

7. Left on Levant.

8. Right on Vulcan Stairway to Ord.

9. Right on Ord to Saturn.

10. Ascend Saturn Stairway to cul-de-sac. Walk to Temple.

11. Left on Temple.

12. Right on 17th St. to Uranus.

13. Cross 17th St. Left on 17th St. to Mars.

14. Right on Mars, and walk on upper level to Corbett.

15. Right on Corbett. Walk on left side to Al's Park. Continue to Clayton.

16. Right at crosswalk into Neighborhood Garden. Ascend stairway to Clayton. Continue right to your beginning.

the stairway. On either side of the center retaining wall and plantings are stairways—one built of railroad ties and the other of concrete. Benches positioned on raised brick and header-board platforms let you sit and enjoy expansive views while nestled in a garden planted with redwood, *Acanthus,* privet shrubs, and *Agapanthus.*

◢ At the top of the stairs, you enter a cul-de-sac of Saturn, a divided street where you walk along the upper level, and then you ascend short stairways on the walkway to Temple. The houses are small.

◢ Turn left on Temple. At 17th St. turn right, heading uphill to Uranus. Cross at the stoplight here, and double-back (left) on 17th St. to Mars. With the 17% grade on this thoroughfare, you can appreciate the difference stairways make in navigating hills. The small section on the south side of 17th St. will help you appreciate the land contours and lets you walk by some older homes and cottages, which have been

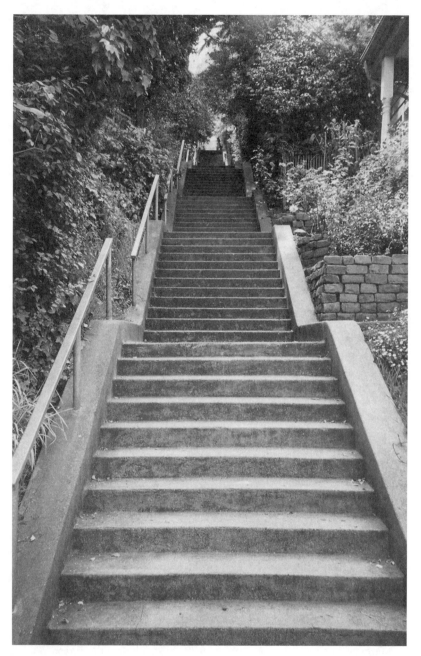

Vulcan Stairway   *Peter Nagy*

here since the 1880s. This area is part of the Eureka Valley neighborhood, which has one of the oldest functioning community organizations in the city. During the 1980s, there was extensive renovation of the Victorian homes here.

◢ Turn right on Mars, and walk on the upper side. Continue to Corbett, turn right, and on the left-hand side next to No. 377 is Al's Park, which extends to Market. Al has been taking care of his park for many years and has been most generous in distributing the fruits of his labor. The park contains fountains, flowers, benches, and fruit trees; the apples are wonderful!

◢ Bearing right, you reach Clayton. (In the first decade of the 20th century, this was the site of the Mountain House Inn. A wood bridge here covered a runoff originating from Mountain Springs.) Turn right at the crosswalk, and cross to the flourishing Neighborhood Garden (see Walk 17) that has been an active volunteer effort since 1960.

◢ Ascend the stairway in the garden to Clayton, and turn right. Market is below and the Mt. Sutro TV Tower is to the left. Don't forget to look back. Continue on Clayton to 17th St. to your beginning. Walk on the right side for Bay views.

Further Rambling

If you wish to link this walk with the one for Twin Peaks Foothills, from the end point of this walk, follow the directions for Walk 17, starting with Steps 7–15, and then follow Steps 1–6.

You can also step into the nearby wilderness of the Sutro Urban Forest. Trails and stairways there connect with the Cole Valley and Upper Haight neighborhoods. Walk four blocks north on 17th St. to Stanyan from Clayton. Cross the street carefully, watching for traffic. Enter where a sign reads, "QUIET, up to the Forest"—there is a lot to see.

Trees, Rocks & Underground Wiring

Corona Heights

This walk takes you to both sides of Corona Heights, which is bounded roughly by Roosevelt, 15th St., States St., and Castro. From here you have easy access to the neighborhoods lying south of Market, via Castro and Clayton. Corona Heights was once an enclave of Hollywood silent-film stars, including Rudolph Valentino and Norma Talmadge, along with local sugar barons like the Spreckels family. The Corona Heights neighborhood offers much to discover presently, in addition to its history.

The walk itself has the richness and variety of a satisfying meal. The setting is complex. To the west you see the dramatic rock formation of Corona Hill (510 feet), geologically part of the Franciscan Formation and very near the city's geographical center. To the east, you see hills, high-rises, and the Bay. Within the neighborhood, you see the shapes and textures of the street trees and individual gardens, Edwardian houses ornamented with varied architectural details and painted in appealing color combinations, small businesses at street level that provide services and goods for everyday needs (laundries, cleaners, coffeehouses, grocery stores, and hardware stores), and a sky unblemished by overhead electrical wires.

The Randall Museum is also a popular educational site for people of all ages. Currently the museum presents lectures, has exhibits on geology and anthropology, and offers classes in natural history, photography, ceramics, and carpentry. It also houses an important collection of live native animals, the subject of one of their most popular talk series. (The museum welcomes volunteers. For more information, call 415-554-9600.)

WALK FACTS

The Eureka Valley MUNI Station, which is the eastern end of the Twin Peaks Tunnel that you take to reach the West Portal Station, is still visible above Market and Castro, but it closed in 1972; its entrance on the north side of Market just above Castro Street looks maintenance related, but it was kept open for emergencies after the Castro Station opened in 1980.

Corona Heights has also been known as Rock Hill, Rocky Hill, and even Randall Hill. The city purchased the land that was once the Gray Brothers quarry and brick factory in 1928, and the park was renamed Corona Heights in 1941.

The Randall Museum houses traveling and permanent science exhibits. A popular one worth noting is their earthquake exhibit, which features a seismograph recording of earthquake action in the area, and the seismometer allows you to feel the intensity of the registered earthquake. The Randall Museum is open Tuesday–Saturday, 10 a.m.–5 p.m.

Bus Routes & Parking

PUBLIC TRANSPORTATION: MUNI Bus #37 Corbett. Several Metro Lines stop at the Castro Street Station. For MUNI bus or Metro information, call 311 (outside San Francisco, call 415-701-2311).

PARKING: There is metered street parking available; metered parking is usually available for up to an hour, and free street parking is usually allowed for up to two hours. But also look for street-cleaning times posted in the neighborhood to avoid getting ticketed or towed.

WALK 19 DESCRIPTION

◢ Begin at the intersection of Buena Vista Terrace and Roosevelt Way. Walking downhill on the odd-numbered side of Roosevelt, you face the Bay. Behind you is the large, handsome structure that was St. Joseph's Hospital and is now the 220-unit Park Hill Condominiums.

◢ Across the street from No. 26 Roosevelt and next to No. 75, which has a tile plaque of the 16th-century fortified tower in Portugal known as Torre de Belem on the right side of the doorway, is the Henry Stairway. Descend the Henry Stairway to the cul-de-sac. Bottlebrush trees delineate the entrance. Two flat false-front Italianates—No. 215 (1906) and No. 213 (1905)—and a pitched-roof with a bay at No. 209 (1906) are of particular interest on this block of Henry.

◢ The hillside continues to be tended by neighbors in the cul-de-sac. To your left is the back of McKinley School, a two-story building. The long and wide trompe l'oeil stairway from the playground up to the classrooms, painted in a variety of colors vertically divided, gives the illusion of a painting. The surrounding walls are decorated with figures, flowers, and words.

◢ Cross Castro at the stoplight (where it's safer) one block to the left at 14th St. There is also a fine corner grocery where you can buy trail nourishment.

◢ Go back to Henry, and turn left. Nos. 195–193 have protruding wires along the edge of the porch roof to prevent pigeons from roosting there.

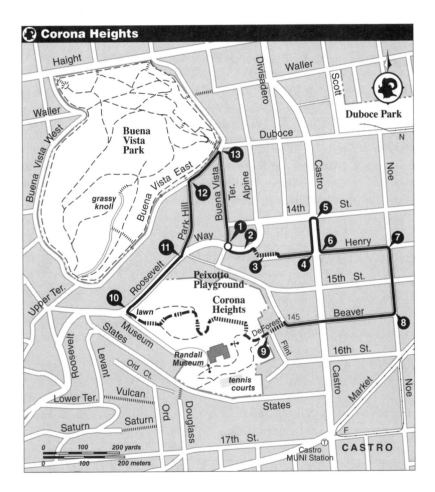

QUICK-STEP INSTRUCTIONS

1. Begin at Roosevelt Way and Buena Vista Terrace.

2. Walk downhill on odd-numbered side of Roosevelt.

3. Descend Henry Stairway at No. 473 Roosevelt and continue to Castro.

4. Left to 14th St. Cross Castro.

5. Return to Henry St.

6. Left on Henry to Noe.

7. Right on Noe to Beaver.

8. Right on Beaver. Next to No. 145 Beaver, ascend DeForest Stairway into Corona Park.

9. Follow path and stairways to Roosevelt.

10. Right on Roosevelt to Park Hill.

11. Left on Park Hill to Buena Vista East.

12. Right on Buena Vista East to Buena Vista Terrace.

13. Right on Buena Vista Terrace to your beginning.

◢ Turn right on Noe. The first block is particularly likeable; it reflects a village ambiance reminiscent of a New York City neighborhood like Sutton Place. A strong sense of nature pervades the street. The green canopies of ficus, carob, gingko, London plane trees, and eucalyptus, together with the variegated colors of impatiens, fuchsias, daisies, and camellias planted in boxes around small shrubs, create a flourishing environment around the small stores.

◢ Cross 15th St., and continue to the mini-community garden park at the corner of Noe and Beaver, a felicitous space for friends and neighbors to meet and visit. Turn right on Beaver, where the synergistic effect of a fine assortment of Stick-style Italianates and street trees continues. You are walking uphill. Cross Castro at 16th St. (where it's safer), and continue upward on Beaver. There is an attractive two-family home and adjoining garden at Nos. 123–125 Beaver (1879) set back from the street. And next to No. 145 Beaver lies the lovely DeForest Stairway.

◢ Before ascending DeForest, you may want to look at the unusual wall of polished chert slickensides across from No. 174 Beaver. As you walk around it (Peixotto Playground is to your right), you see the best example in the city of these geologically smoothed rock faces. The term *slickensides* evokes just the right way of describing the feel of the stone against your skin. Be sure to rub your hands over the cold, smooth, shiny surfaces, the result of rock grinding against rock under terrifically high pressure for millions of years.

◢ Ascend the stairway to the top, where you'll be at the tennis courts of Corona Heights Park. Walk through the gate, and bear right immediately as you go uphill. Stop for a moment to turn around and look at the Bay, just visible between the buildings to the east.

◢ You are now in back of the Randall Museum, commonly known as the Junior Museum. Located at No. 199 Museum Way, the museum is positioned within one of the most scenic topographical areas in the city—an assemblage of 140-million- to 160-million-year-old chert and sandstone. The Randall Museum is dedicated to Josephine Randall, the first superintendent of recreation in San Francisco. She was able to fulfill her dream of establishing a nature museum, which to this day instills in children and adults a love of science, natural history, and the arts. It moved to its present location in 1951.

◢ At the fork in the path where the eucalyptus tree stands, bear right on the stairway. The tree was planted in 1990 to minimize erosion of the fragile hill, while also giving young native plants the opportunity to take root. Plant-restoration work parties are an ongoing monthly volunteer activity.

◢ Ahead of you now is the startlingly beautiful and ever-expanding panoramic view of the Bay and the hills below you. Downtown San Francisco lies to the north, and Bernal Heights, crowned at its summit with a microwave power station, lies to the south. To your left, you can see McKinley Elementary School below, striking with its blue-trimmed vents and contrasting bright red roof. Here you can get a sense of Corona Hill's height, while watching rock climbers practice their craft. Nearby find a conveniently placed bench, which also makes a perfect station for full-moon viewing; plan to visit this spot for a Harvest Moon if possible.

◢ To the right at the next landing, you can see the 220-unit Park Hill Condominiums with its distinctive terra-cotta tile roof. Continue up the short stairway to the left, and walk to the signpost stating "Summit 150 Ft." Follow the stairways to the top for a 360-degree view.

In 1881 Dr. Ed Livingstone Trudeau walked the length of Manhattan—from Central Park to the Battery—in 47 minutes on a bet.

⊿ From the opposite side of the summit, descend the stairways and path that leads into a clearing adjacent to a dog run. One of the amenities of the dog run is a doggie water fountain. Exit at the gate near the sign that reads "Randall Museum."

⊿ You're now at Museum Way and Roosevelt. If you would like to visit the museum, go left on Museum Way for a short distance. The Randall Museum, including the gates to the gardens and the walkway to the front entrance, is designed with incised replicas of plants and flowers.

⊿ When you are ready, return to Roosevelt, and turn right. There is an attractive array of varied architecture on this street from the redwood shingle tuck-in at No. 284 Roosevelt (1907) to the row of Queen Annes: No. 227 (1900) and Nos. 225 and 223 (1903). The newer town houses across the street and farther down are consonant with the ambiance of the block. In addition, their exterior colors contribute softness and sparkle to the street.

⊿ Continue on Roosevelt to Park Hill, and turn left. No. 77 has both a living arbor front door entrance and a living fence.

McKinley Playground   *Adah Bakalinsky*

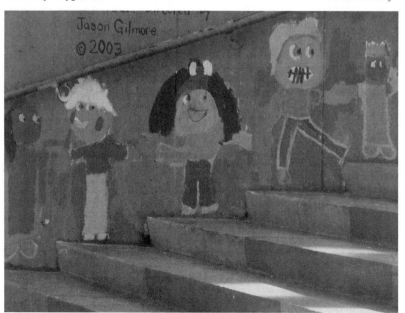

◢ At Buena Vista East, turn left to see the aesthetic Park Hill condos. The front door and back large glass windows are aligned so that the panoramic view through the back is reflected in the front.

◢ Buena Vista Park, across the street, was designated as a park in 1870, the same year as Golden Gate Park. It has paths, benches, many trees, various elevations, and many wood stairways. The extensive renovation to curb erosion-control and reforest the park, along with all the new stairs and walkways added to the south and southwest side make it worthy of its name, which means "good view." (If you have time, amble through now. Or, better yet, take Walk 30, Upper Haight, and circumambulate the Adah Bakalinsky Stairway at the beginning.) As Adah always says, "I heartily recommend you make a special excursion to explore the park."

◢ Return to the corner of Park Hill to continue along Buena Vista East. No. 181, at the corner of Buena Vista East and Duboce, is an imposing structure on an acre of land with extensive gardens in back. Once occupied by US Ambassador James Hormel and known as the Hormel Mansion, this Queen Anne and lot could legally be divided into five lots. But fortunately, an individual who purchased the house in 2007 intends to keep it as a one-family unit.

◢ At the grand entrance to Buena Vista Park, turn right on Buena Vista Terrace. Walk past 14th St. and back to your beginning.

Further Rambling

Now that you've had the grand excursion around the park, take another grand amble by linking to Walk 30, which takes you up into Buena Vista Park and visits the Adah Bakalinsky Stairway. The Upper Haight neighborhood retains a shopping district along Haight St. up to Stanyan and Golden Gate Park, just a few more blocks west.

Or if you'd prefer to walk downhill from here, visit the Lower Haight by walking one block north to Haight St., and head downhill. The Upper and Lower Haight St. neighborhoods are mainly divided at Divisadero.

Amazing Footpaths

Eureka Valley

Eureka Valley encompasses the area below the southeastern slope of Twin Peaks. Wedged between Diamond Heights, Noe Valley, and Upper Market, it has one of the oldest, continuously functioning neighborhood associations in the city. In the 1920s, the neighborhood was mostly Scandinavian and Irish. The Swedish church was on Dolores St.; the Scandinavian deli, on Market. John Nurmi's bar at No. 258 Noe was a great gathering place for the Finnish residents. Schubert's Bakery on Market employed 10 bakers and was famous citywide for its excellent pastries. Joseph Affolter's father moved his butcher shop to No. 2283 Market in 1930 because he wanted the overflow of customers from the bakery. After he retired, his four sons operated the butcher shop for more than 50 years until their deaths. The sign on the wall said, "Don't swear. Smile." When Adah spoke to him, Joseph recalled that all the meat, including the beef stew, was sold with bone in it, and the fillet was part of the sirloin and tenderloin cuts. Families used to shop for meat and fish twice a day.

Eureka Valley's Castro St. (now known as the Castro neighborhood) is the shopping center and hub of the gay community, an important sociological and political force in San Francisco since 1970. In 1977, Harvey Milk became the first openly gay member of the San Francisco Board of Supervisors. (His photography shop and campaign headquarters at Nos. 573–575 Castro is now City Landmark No. 227.) Milk and Mayor George Moscone were murdered in City Hall in November 1978 by Dan White, a deranged former supervisor. Harry Britt was appointed to Milk's former position as an openly gay supervisor. The gay rights movement's outspokenness, fervor, and passion created an awareness among the general public of discrimination against gays and lesbians in the San Francisco Police Department and in the workplace; it also influenced the Board of Supervisors to pass San Francisco's domestic partners law, which provides health insurance benefits to partners of gay city employees.

(Continued on page 172)

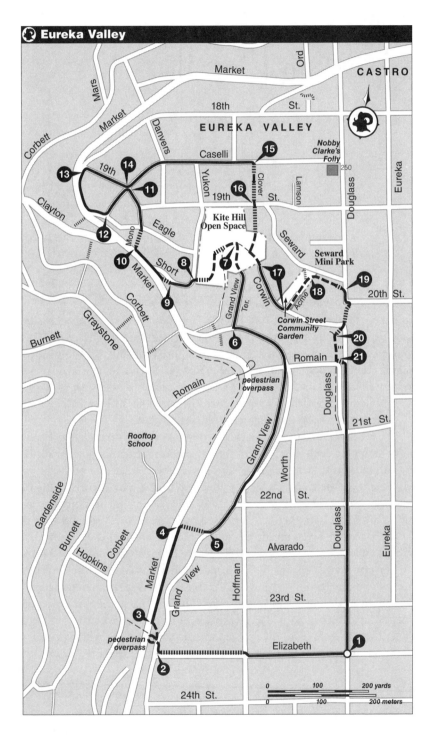

QUICK-STEP INSTRUCTIONS

1. Begin at Elizabeth and Douglass. Walk one block on the right-hand side of Elizabeth to Hoffman. Ascend the sidewalk stairway to Grand View.

2. Cross Grand View, and walk on pedestrian overpass to Market.

3. Right on Market.

4. Right on Dixie Stairway (next to No. 3801 Market) to Grand View (across from No. 285).

5. Left on Grand View. Continue on the upper side to Grand View Terrace.

6. Right on Grand View Terrace to enter Kite Hill Open Space.

7. Bear left on second footpath and railroad-tie stairway down to Yukon between Short and Eagle.

8. Left on Yukon to Short. Bear right and ascend Short Stairway to Market.

9. Right on Market.

10. Right on Mono Stairway to Eagle. Cross Eagle to continue on Mono right-of-way to 19th St.

11. Veer left on 19th St. to Caselli. Left on Caselli.

12. Right on Eagle to Market. Turn right onto Market.

13. Right on 19th St., facing Kite Hill.

14. Left on Caselli.

15. Next to No. 101 Caselli, ascend Clover Lane Stairway to 19th St.

16. Cross 19th St. and continue up the stairway, next to No. 4615, onto a dirt path on the north side of Kite Hill.

17. Follow the left path leading into Corwin, and walk to Corwin Street Community Garden on the left side of the street opposite No. 95. Walk down the (Acme Alley) driveway beside the garden to Seward Mini Park opposite No. 30 Seward.

18. Right on upper pedestrian walkway of Seward. Descend stairway to Douglass.

19. Right on Douglass to 20th. Ascend Douglass Stairway. Cross Corwin and ascend stairway.

20. Walk on pedestrian walkway of Douglass (right side) to Romain.

21. Descend stairway, and continue on Douglass to Elizabeth to your beginning.

(Continued from page 169)

The Castro neighborhood supports a variety of boutiques, stores, restaurants, and bars. And the crown jewel of the Castro is the historic landmark Castro Theatre. Their programming includes revivals of American and foreign films and special events, such as the Lesbian and Gay, Jewish, and Silent Film Festivals. Every evening an organist plays the Wurlitzer before the first show. David Hegarty accompanies the silent features and also plays for the San Francisco Legion of Honor. Timothy Pfleuger designed the 1922 Spanish Renaissance–style movie palace, as well as the former Pacific Exchange (now an Equinox Fitness Center), 450 Sutter Building, and the Paramount Theatre in Oakland.

The gay influence on the neighborhood is apparent in many facets of street life: the rainbow banners attached to the light standards, the many skillful renovations of Victorian homes throughout the neighborhood, the generally available taxis due to the abundance of street traffic, people carrying bouquets of flowers as gifts or for their homes, and the great shops and watering holes like the Twin Peaks Tavern at Market (enduring and highly visible for more than 30 years) and the popular Cliff's Hardware store (one of the best of its kind in San Francisco). This neighborhood, even when it is crowded for a film festival, or other special events and holidays, still maintains its friendly, kind, and courteous outlook and is quite enjoyable to visit.

More strenuous than some, this walk has an eloquent cadence of many kinds of stairways; paths, alleyways, and skyways; unusual gardens; tree-lined streets; open spaces; and houses with special architectural details. The area remains visually interesting through many repeated strolls. Views from it are exceptional. Bring binoculars and perhaps an orange or two (to boost your energy).

WALK FACTS

Although it stays above the Castro District, this walk moves through streets that were the scene of great strife and turf warfare concerning water. Unfortunately, the natural springs under Twin Peaks were destroyed when tunnel work began in 1914.

Events in the Castro District run the gamut from healthy, outdoor, kid-friendly options to nightly more adult-themed burlesque parties and bar scenes. The nearby Eureka Valley Recreation Center offers classes to anyone who would like to join. St. Phillips Church hosts historical talks, and Harvey's hosts free comedy shows on

Tuesdays. Plus, the many dance parties and stage shows put on by local entertainers and barkeeps here can either keep you on your feet, or knock you off your feet, depending on your interests.

Bus Routes & Parking

PUBLIC TRANSPORTATION: MUNI Bus #48 Quintara and #24 Divisadero. Several Metro lines stop at the Castro Street Station, much farther away. For MUNI bus information, call 311 (outside San Francisco, call 415-701-2311).

PARKING: There is metered street parking available; metered parking is usually available for up to an hour, and free street parking is usually allowed for up to two hours. But also look for street-cleaning times posted in the neighborhood to avoid getting ticketed or towed.

WALK 20 DESCRIPTION

◢ Begin at Elizabeth and Douglass, and walk west on the right-hand side of Elizabeth. You are gradually walking uphill—a perfect introduction to the sidewalk stairway that begins at Hoffman. Abundant and diverse vegetation grows on both sides of the street. Several homeowners decided to put in garages on Elizabeth that cut into the previously long, uninterrupted stairway. The residents of No. 966 display a garden of disarming combinations of colors and textures. After crossing Grand View, bear right to the pedestrian overpass above Market, where you have a wondrous view of the eastern half of the city.

◢ Turn right on Market. At No. 3801 turn right onto the Dixie Stairway, and descend to Grand View.

◢ Continue to the left on Grand View. At 22nd St., walk on the left side on upper Grand View where you'll see a curly leaf willow growing. Walk past Romain along this divided street.

◢ Make a right turn on Grand View Terrace, which leads to the Kite Hill Open Space. Purchased with open-space funds in 1976, Kite Hill is inviting and functional. Walkers use it, as do dogs and their owners. Kite Hill was once owned by "Nobby" Clarke's Water Works and then the Spring Valley Water Works (then Company), and it was also once known as Solari Hill for a farmer who let his cattle graze there before the spring was commercialized. But in 1976, thanks to neighbors led by Doris Murphy, the public rallied to have San Francisco purchase the land and turn it into a park.

- On the Yukon slope of Kite Hill (facing 19th St.), the Natural Areas Program of the Recreation and Parks Department has restored native plants to the area, including gooseberry (*Ribes*), footsteps of spring (*Sanicula arctopoides*), and wild parsley (*Lomatium dasycarpum*), a favorite of the anise swallowtail butterfly, along with California buttercup (*Ranunculus californicus*), California aster (*Aster chilensis*), and California brome grass (*Bromus californica*). From the top of the hill, there's a triangular configuration of open-space areas: Tank Hill to the left, Corona Heights to the right, and Kite Hill, where you stand, at the top of the triangle.

- At the corner of Yukon and 19th St., at the base of the open-space area, a resident has planted a flourishing garden of ginger, *Echium,* and *Euphorbia,* which is contrary to the native-species restoration of this area, but not too intrusively so, as their spiky red, purple, and yellow forms rise up as if they've been native to the area for millions of years.

- Bear left on the second footpath, and take the railroad-tie stairway to Yukon between Eagle and Short. Turn left, walk across to Short, bear right, and continue past valerian and nasturtium growing along the retaining wall. Ascend Short Stairway to Market, turn right, and continue to Mono Stairway.

- Turn right on Mono Stairway to Eagle. Growing alongside are lantana, *Ceanothus,* and rock rose, which have white petals with red targets that indicate the route to the nectar. Cross Eagle to continue to 19th St. on the Mono right-of-way, with its archaeological paving mix, consisting of new and old brick bound with concrete. Here, at the end of Mono, a neighbor has turned an unused city lot into a veritable Shangri-La. The David Austin roses not only look magnificent planted, but their aroma is heavenly; they will root you to the spot. At least 30 varieties of birds come here to feed and sing.

- Turn left on 19th St. and left again onto Caselli. Near No. 312 Caselli the street is plainly still edged with cobblestone.

- Turn right on Eagle and then right on Market. Market Street was originally named Falcon Road, and later, it transformed again into a toll road named Corbett (part of Corbett still remains). Market did not exist west of Eureka until the 1920s. Yet this thoroughfare over to the Parkside development that came to be known as the Sunset, Richmond, Mount Davidson, and Forest Hill became more and more important as the city expanded out to the west throughout the 1920s to the 1940s. Between 1956 and 1958, Market had become such an important arterial road that it was widened to four lanes. Usually Market Street is a thoroughfare you drive, so walking here reveals a trove of unsuspected architecture and gardens.

⚓ On the hill across the street, at No. 3224, is a large pink house (two smaller ones are later additions) on a 90-foot-deep lot. Known as the Miller-Joost House, it was built in 1867 by Adam Miller, a German immigrant, carpenter, and dairy rancher. Miller's daughter, Anna, and her husband, Behrend Joost, occupied this house after they married. Behrend, who built the first electric railroad from Steuart and Market to the county line in Colma, later also owned the local Mountain Springs Water Company until the Twin Peaks Tunnel excavation disrupted its flow. The Miller-Joost House has attained landmark status (Landmark 79). (If this piques your interest, see the Further Rambling section at the end of this walk.) One of my favorite murals, which I call the "Landscape of San Francisco," by Betsie Miller-Kusz, runs along on the wall below the Miller-Joost House on Market St.

⚓ Turn right on 19th St., where you will be facing Kite Hill. Turn left on Caselli. At the corner of Danvers, a former church is now a private home.

⚓ Next to No. 101 Caselli, on the right side of the street, ascend the Clover Lane Stairway to 19th St. The walkway here is reminiscent of an old-fashioned alley in Chicago. Near No. 4612 19th St. (at the top of the stairway) cross the street, and continue up the stairway beside No. 4615. The dirt section above this stairway leads to the north side of Kite Hill.

⚓ A bench here is perfect for contemplating a panoramic view of the Bay Bridge. Walk to your left to take in a view of Corona Heights and the downtown skyline, with Eureka Valley and the US Mint in the foreground. Also after a respite on the bench, follow the path right that you can see branching into Corwin. Across the street is the remarkable Corwin Street Community Garden. Adah and I have both been very fortunate to witness the metamorphosis of this land since 1995. The signage is excellent; the choice of vegetation is botanically superior. Butterflies and birds use this garden, and in return, they buzz, pollinate, warble, and sing in thanks. Among the beds of 67 native flowers, shrubs, and trees attractive to butterflies and hummingbirds are yarrow, mimulus, coyote bush, and mallow. Because of the sit-in staged in 1966 to save this parcel of land from being developed, San Francisco changed the way it approached development, and legislation that came out of this community protest requires open-space planning to be part of all neighborhood development projects.

Mary Walker, 82, of Philadelphia became a walker during a transit strike. For years, she had held down a full-time job at one of the nation's largest banks. After work each day, she put on her sneakers and took the 7.5-mile walk home. She enjoyed every bit of the walk and saw people racing by, which was not her style. As she explained, "I get home when I get home."

◢ Walk down the condo driveway, Acme Alley, a cobblestone thruway running alongside the garden entrance to Seward Mini Park. With the added benefit of being protected from the wind, it's a fine setting for a picnic lunch. In the early days of San Francisco, Acme Alley was the path used to take cattle from Mission Dolores to pasture.

◢ Turn right on upper Seward. This elevated pedestrian walkway gives you a better view of neighborhood gardens. Continue on this walkway, and descend the stairway to Douglass.

◢ Turn right to 20th St. and right to ascend the Douglass Stairway. At the top, look back at the view of Corona Heights Hill. Cross Corwin, and ascend the stairway to the upper level of divided Douglass to enjoy a better view.

◢ Descend the stairway at Romain to Douglass. The Alvarado Elementary School at No. 625 Douglass (at the corner of 22nd St.) has a mural flanking its entrance, in memory of two wonderful teachers. Through the initiative and leadership of sculptor Ruth Asawa, the school has had an enrichment art program for more than four decades. Asawa used children's art for her public fountains in the Hyatt hotel courtyard and in Ghirardelli Square. Her son and daughter have continued the Asawa family tradition, which has become a community legacy.

◢ The school walls and fence are painted with city scenes and water scenes. One section of the fence is decorated with painted mosaic tiles of a school, a bus, and children's heads in a tree. Assembled on the outer side of a wall of the playground is a 42-foot by 11-foot ceramic mural with a theme of nature and gardening that is dedicated to Ruth Asawa. It was completed in May 2000, a two-year project in which students, teachers, and artists participated. In 2010,

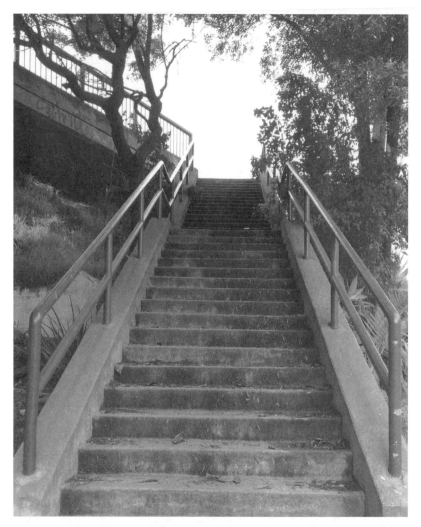

Short Street Stairway   *Mary Burk*

the School of the Arts High School was renamed the Ruth Asawa San Francisco School of Arts.

◢ At the corner of 23rd St. are five false-gable, rectangular-bay homes to your left. From the middle of the street looking west (in line with the middle of Twin Peaks), you might recall Daniel Burnham's plan for a magnificent view corridor from the Ferry Building to Twin Peaks. The 1906 earthquake and subsequent hurried rebuilding of the town, though, prevented his 1905 plan, called the San Francisco City

Beautiful plan, from being implemented. However, some neighborhoods partly followed the Burnham plan, and Walks 12 (St. Francis Wood) and 15 (Forest Hill), built after the earthquake and fire, showcase the elegance of that design.

◢ Turn toward Elizabeth St. and back to your beginning.

Further Rambling

"Nobby" Clarke's Folly at No. 250 Douglass (at the corner of Caselli) is a king-sized Queen Anne mansion with landmark status. Built on a 17-acre lot in 1892 for $100,000, the five-story mansion had 45 rooms, 52 closets, 10 fireplaces, and 272 windows. It has since been converted to 15 one-bedroom apartments.

Clarke was an Irish sailor who immigrated to California in 1850. Beginning his career as a gold miner, he later worked in the police department, became a lawyer, and finally pursued a career as an entrepreneur. The springs flowing from Joost's property in upper Twin Peaks followed the north side of Caselli to Clarke's holdings. Becoming dissatisfied with the service, he started Clarke's Water Works, but in 1896 he went bankrupt. It's worth walking over to for a look, perhaps before taking in a nice matinee.

Corwin Stairway   *Mary Burk*

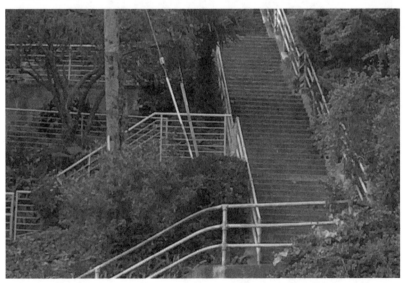

A Mondrian Walk

Dolores Heights

A good walk is an organism of mysterious nuances that can affect us in subtle ways, from quiet harmoniousness to ebullience, from languor to exuberance. Within a stroll for a stamp, a loaf of bread, a bit of exercise, or a breath of fresh air are the promising ingredients of an imaginative walk that charms and delights: the various terrain to traverse, the spectrum of colors to see in the sky, the views of manufactured objects to comprehend, the assortment of people to meet, and even the intrinsic rhythm and shape of the walk to sense, as you feel it out, or discover it as you go.

Adah explained to me how she loves to trace out the shape of a walk on paper after walking it. This exercise shows her if there is a correlation between its shape and how it feels. On this walk, she may have found a new correlation in shapes. To illustrate the concept, some of Adah's early walks usually took on the shape of a foot or a shoe, and she described them as feeling very comfortable. Later walks took on new shapes, forming fanciful figures and even geometric patterns like this one, and yet, they felt effortless. This walk through Dolores Heights is a Mondrian choreography, a study in working urban forms leading you on easily to your next gorgeous destination.

WALK FACTS

Nearby sidewalks need steps cut into them, just above Dolores Park at 22nd Street (between Church and Vicksburg), and the street has a 31.5% grade, tying it for first with Filbert (between Leavenworth and Hyde) as being the steepest street in San Francisco.

Close by Noe Valley was originally named Horner's Addition, because John Horner had purchased the land divided out of Rancho San Miguel. But in 1857 a stock market crash wiped out Horner, forcing him to mortgage all of his San Francisco real estate to pay off debt.

On this side of Twin Peaks, sunny weather is more common than it is in the western part of the city. Watch for late afternoon westerly winds to blow clouds over Twin Peaks; they move so quickly that they may appear to be in high-speed motion.

Bus Routes & Parking

PUBLIC TRANSPORTATION: MUNI Bus #33 Stanyan and Metro J Church. For MUNI bus or Metro information, call 311 (outside San Francisco, call 415-701-2311).

PARKING: There is metered street parking available; metered parking is usually available for up to an hour, and free street parking is usually allowed for up to two hours. But also look for street-cleaning times posted in the neighborhood to avoid getting ticketed or towed.

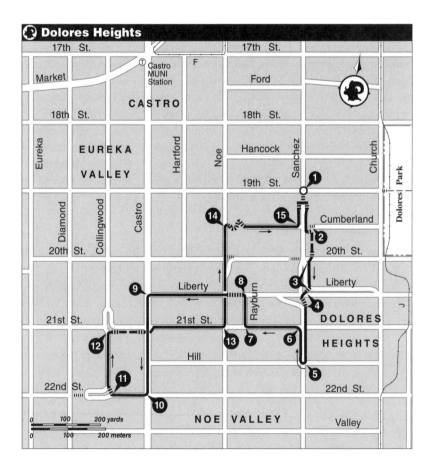

QUICK-STEP INSTRUCTIONS

1. Begin at 19th St. and Sanchez. Ascend Sanchez Stairway to Cumberland.

2. At No. 655 Sanchez, descend small stairway. Turn right onto pedestrian walkway to 20th St.

3. Continue on left side onto lower Sanchez. Ascend stairway to Liberty.

4. Cross Liberty to ascend Sanchez Stairway. Continue past 21st St. to Hill St.

5. Loop back on Sanchez to 21st St.

6. Left on 21st St., and walk to Rayburn.

7. Right on Rayburn, and walk to Liberty.

8. Left on Liberty. Descend stairway to Noe. Continue to Castro.

9. Left on Castro to 22nd St.

10. Right on 22nd St.

11. Right and ascend stairway to Collingwood. Walk to 21st St.

12. Right on 21st St. Descend sidewalk stairway. Continue past Castro to Noe.

13. Left on Noe to Cumberland Stairway across from No. 670 Noe.

14. Right to ascend Cumberland Stairway. Continue to Sanchez.

15. Left on Sanchez. Descend Sanchez Stairway to 19th St. and your beginning.

WALK 21 DESCRIPTION

◢ Begin at 19th St. and Sanchez. California lilacs (*Ceanothus*), bottle-brush, and acacia grow at the base of the imposing wall flanking the double stairways going up Sanchez. (The first City inspection recorded on the stairways is from 1939.) Ascend the left stairway. A contemporary home at the top, No. 615 Sanchez, has replaced a small house that once stood here. The four cypress trees in front of the house are more than a half century old. At one time Sanchez had brick paving, but the brick was too slick and had to be covered with asphalt.

◢ The intersection of Cumberland and Sanchez is a special corner for its combination of houses and trees, a feeling of neighborliness that pervades the street, the configuration of the two streets affording both close-up and distant views, and the surprise of seeing all this at the end of the first ascent of this route.

⌐ Continue walking on Sanchez. A few feet farther on, you can see the section of the Cumberland Stairway that goes down to Church. At No. 650 Sanchez (at Cumberland), cape jasmine and trumpet vine grow under the veranda. Penstemon, valerian, mimulus, rosemary, and *Acanthus* brighten the block. Continue walking on the left (east) side of Sanchez. At Cumberland, the dome of the Christian Science Temple on Dolores is visible.

⌐ In front of No. 655 Sanchez, descend the stairs to the pedestrian walkway. Go to your right. At No. 674 Sanchez, New Zealand flax grows behind the rock. You're walking south toward 20th St. on the east side of the street. A center strip of flora and unusual, tilted stairs divide the upper and lower parts of Sanchez between 20th St. and Liberty. Continue walking on the left side of lower Sanchez. Ascend the stairway to Liberty.

⌐ Cross Liberty to continue up the Sanchez Stairway, which is fronted by a high retaining wall. The redwood-shingled house, No. 746 Sanchez, conforms to the irregularly shaped lot in a comfortable way; it stretches around the corner. The off-center arched veranda (or maybe it is a carport, but there is a garage off to the side) leads the eye to the terraced garden, where camellias and a mature Douglas-fir are the dominant plants.

Sanchez Stairway   *Adah Bakalinsky*

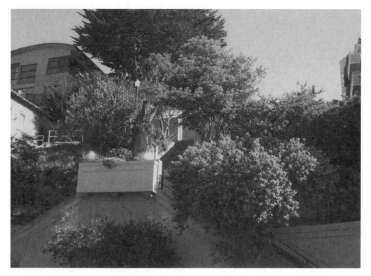

- Continue to 21st St. The house at the corner, No. 3690, formerly belonged to James "Sunny Jim" Rolph Jr., the popular San Francisco mayor (1912–1931). John McLaren, who was the superintendent of Golden Gate Park for 60 years, planted the Monterey pine trees around the house. At No. 3701 21st St., a sculptured redwood bench is inset on tile and dedicated to Audrey Penn Rodgers by friends, relatives, and neighbors. She was president of the Dolores Heights Improvement Club for many years and diligently watched over the area to make sure it retained its unique neighborhood ambiance.

The swiftest traveler is he that goes afoot. —Henry David Thoreau

- Walk toward Hill, formerly called "Nanny Goat Hill" in reference to the goats that grazed here, and enjoy the view to the south. At the turn of the century, the designated neighborhood voting place was a small structure on the top of the hill (right). Before the streets were paved, firefighters, who worked at the 22nd St. firehouse between Sanchez and Noe (now a residence), left their pumps up here on the hill as a kindness to their horses.

- The Native Americans who once lived near Mission Dolores came up here to get their water from the many springs that were in this area. Some houses in the neighborhood still have their own capped wells.

- Historically, working-class people have resided in Dolores Heights, but now many professional people live here, and the mix enriches the neighborhood. The residents love the sunny, fog-free weather.

- At Hill and Sanchez, look left to take in the full measure of the elevation. Retrace your steps on Sanchez to 21st St., and turn left. Turn right on Rayburn, which takes you out to Liberty. After a left turn, you soon reach the Liberty Stairway, which you descend to Noe.

- Four, white, stucco Art Deco houses alongside the stairway are foils for the multitude of neighborhood Victorians, from elaborate Queen Annes of the late 1880s and 1890s to one-story, flat-front Italianates of the 1870s and early 1880s.

- As you walk in the neighborhood, the constantly shifting cloud cover playing with the TV tower on Mt. Sutro, obscuring it one minute and uncovering it the next, can be both captivating and distracting. Be flexible about crossing the street for better views, and mind the traffic around you.

◢ Cross Noe. Walk on the left (south) side of Liberty. The 500 block of Liberty is exquisite, with small and mature trees—London plane, magnolia, and Brisbane box. Nos. 564–576 Liberty were built in 1897 by Fernando Nelson, a prolific developer of tract Victorians in this and other Mission neighborhoods. These houses display his favorite wood embellishments: the decorative circles and pendants that he referred to as "donuts" and "drips."

◢ Continue on Liberty to Castro. Corona Heights, previously known as Rock Hill, comes into view. Turn left on Castro. Queen Anne row houses are on the even-numbered side of the 700 block of Castro. (Look for the donuts and drips.)

◢ Walk to 22nd St. and turn right. This section of 22nd St. is a turnabout; a sculptural, high-curved retaining wall encompasses the stairway you now ascend to Collingwood. (The stairway beyond it goes down to Diamond.) You're at the top of the hill of this five-block street.

◢ Turn right on Collingwood. In 1932, a German mason built the cobblestone house at No. 480 out of stones from the dismantled Castro cable car line. Turn right on 21st St., which used to be extremely steep from Diamond to Castro. In 1924 the city "improved" the street by lowering the grade on one side while raising it on the other, resulting in a grade-separated street and some nonfunctioning garages. The one at No. 3937 was converted into living space.

◢ Walk down the sidewalk stairway on the odd-numbered side of 21st St., and continue to Noe. The 3800 block of 21st St. has an exceptional row of Queen Anne Victorians. On the left side, they gently follow the slope of the hill. John Anderson, a contractor, built Nos. 3836–3616 in 1903 and 1904. Your view from here includes the top third of the Mount Sutro TV Tower.

◢ Turn left on Noe. At Liberty, look right to see the stairway you previously descended. From No. 741 (on the odd-numbered side of Noe), you can see the skyline to the north and west. Continue on Noe past the curved retaining wall of 20th St. and the narrow stairway alongside the apartment house at No. 695. The houses on the even-numbered side of the street could become a showcase like those on Alamo Square, or on Clay across from Alta Plaza Park. Three-quarters of the ubiquitous TV tower is still in sight.

◢ Ascend the Cumberland Stairway across from No. 670 Noe. The retaining wall, made from cobblestones, is a backdrop to the rock outcropping upon which the stairway was built. Several century plants, set into the rock soil, form a strong upright profile against the jumbled Franciscan Formation. Sedum, gazanias, and ivy grow here and there.

◢ From the cul-de-sac entrance at the top of the stairs, begin a pleasant walk alongside tree-lined houses. The Dolores Heights Special Use District, which runs from Cumberland to part of 22nd St. between Noe and Church, was established in 1980 to provide residential-design guidelines and preserve front gardens. No. 367 has an octagonal belvedere, roofed in a pattern of blue and lavender tiles. On the cobblestone terrace of No. 338 Cumberland, goldfish swim in the pond. The exterior of No. 333 is cement composition board, a relatively new material being used more broadly to prevent mold and moisture damage. The house provides contrast and a contemporary link to the Victorian architecture in the neighborhood. No. 332 is a simple Craftsman-style house.

◢ No. 300 is made up of two 1906 refugee cottages, which were originally located in Dolores Park. Known as bonus-plan cottages, they provided affordable housing to those who lost their homes in the 1906 earthquake and fire. (The Finance Relief, the Red Cross, and the US Army originally funded the project.) The Carpenters Union, Local 22, built 5,610 shacks. In 1997, 17 shacks were still extant.

◢ Continue to Sanchez to arrive at a most splendid corner of Cumberland. Turn left, and descend the Sanchez Stairway to your beginning.

Further Rambling

Places to eat are plentiful along Castro, 18th St., and Market. This walk is not that close to Walk 20 in Eureka Valley to the north or Walk 25 in Fairmount Heights to the south. But you can reach the shopping district areas near both of them fairly quickly. Reach the Castro District by walking two blocks north to 18th St., then turning left and walking west for two blocks up to Castro. Or if you would like to walk around Noe Valley, start your walk back south on Sanchez, and continue to 24th.

From Ship Building Through Dot-Com to Biotech

Potrero Hill

When the Spaniards arrived in the 18th century, the Potrero Hill area was a peninsula with its original shoreline intact. It was also pastureland (*potrero* means "pasture" in Spanish). Horses, cows, and goats grazed the hill during the Spanish and Mexican period. In the latter half of the 19th century, industry located here because of the area's proximity to water. Union Iron Works was one of the largest builders of steel steamships and men-of-war. It later became Bethlehem-Todd. Baker and Hamilton's warehouse was here in 1849; the site is now occupied by Show Place Square and the Galleria Design Center. Tubbs Cordage was in business in 1859, and Tubbs St. is still present and listed on the maps.

Workers for these industries came from Ireland, Scotland, and the Balkans. Irish Hill was located at 22nd St. and Illinois; Scottish shipbuilders mostly lived on Connecticut. In the early 1900s, Greeks and immigrants from Eastern Europe seemed to congregate near Mariposa and Vermont. Molokans, a religious sect composed predominantly of Russian peasants who, in the 1550s, rejected czarist church policy and beliefs of orthodox Christians, settled around Carolina near 20th St. (No. 341 Carolina). There were boardinghouses for workers along Illinois and 3rd St., and cottages along Tennessee cost $585.

Because Potrero Hill was unscathed by the 1906 earthquake and fire, people from destroyed areas migrated here. The tent city, officially Relief Camp No. 10, extended north to Mariposa, south to between 20th and 22nd Sts., west to Indiana, and east to Kentucky (now 3rd St.). In March 1907, the tents could be exchanged for cottages at a cost of $6 per month, and renters could move the cottages to their own lots.

Good weather, good transportation, good views in every direction, and available lots at good prices attracted professionals and artists to the area after World War II. Cooperative community spirit is responsible for the plethora of community gardens, social services available for the elderly and children, and for resolution of long-term environmental problems, such as air pollution from the Pacific Gas & Electric power plants that operated here until March 2011. Trans Bay Cable now provides the city with a new source of electricity from the town of Pittsburg in the East Bay.

Geographically, the Potrero Hill neighborhood is bound by 16th St. to the north, Cesar Chavez to the south, Potrero Ave. to the west, and San Francisco Bay to the east. US Highway 101 to the west and Interstate 280 to the east are additional nearby boundaries that provide easy access to and from other parts of the city. Geologically, Potrero Hill is composed mainly of serpentine rock. At 300 feet in elevation, it commands encompassing views of the city. Climatically, Potrero Hill has some of the best weather in San Francisco because the larger hills to the west shelter it from winds. Sociologically, it is known for its strong sense of community and its ethnically and racially diverse population.

WALK FACTS

Anchor Brewing at De Haro and Mariposa offers free weekday tours that include a beer tasting. Friday tours are booked six months in advance, and other days are booked a couple months out. Anchor has been brewing at this facility since 1977.

When you cross the overpass on US Highway 101 (Step 10), you can visit San Francisco General Hospital, whose brick buildings were dedicated in 1915. It is especially worth a visit when their Frida Kahlo and Diego Rivera paintings are on display (but they are currently on loan to the San Francisco Museum of Modern Art). The deep red of these tallest brick buildings in the city seems to emit radiant heat in the afternoon sun.

Bus Routes & Parking

PUBLIC TRANSPORTATION: MUNI Bus #19 Polk; #22 Fillmore; #10 Townsend; and #48 Quintara. For MUNI bus information, call 311 (outside San Francisco, call 415-701-2311).

PARKING: There is metered street parking available; metered parking is usually available for up to an hour, and free street parking is usually allowed for up to two hours. But also look for street-cleaning times posted in the neighborhood to avoid getting ticketed or towed.

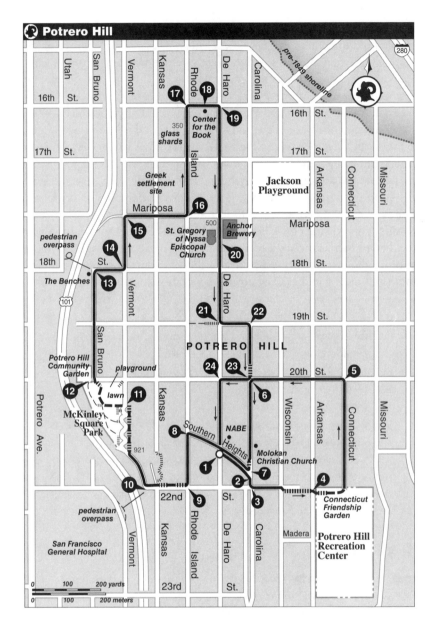

QUICK-STEP INSTRUCTIONS

1. Begin at De Haro and Southern Heights (from Potrero Hill Neighborhood House, or NABE, at No. 953 De Haro).

2. Walk southeast on the curve of Southern Heights to 22nd St.

3. Left on 22nd, and descend 22nd St. Stairway to Arkansas.

4. Cross Arkansas and descend stairway. Continue on path to Connecticut. Left on Connecticut to 20th St.

5. Left on 20th to Carolina.

6. Left on Carolina. Continue to ascend short stairway onto Southern Heights.

7. Curve right on Southern Heights to Rhode Island.

8. Left on Rhode Island to 22nd.

9. Right on 22nd, and descend 22nd St. Stairway. Bear right past Kansas to Vermont.

10. Right on Vermont. At No. 921 Vermont, turn right and ascend stairway. At top of stairway, cross Vermont into McKinley Square Park.

11. Bear left on path around park (past play area). Descend stairway at corner of San Bruno and 20th St.

12. Cross street, and walk along San Bruno to 18th St.

13. Right on 18th St. to Vermont.

14. Left on Vermont to Mariposa.

15. Right on Mariposa to Rhode Island.

16. Left on Rhode Island to No. 350.

17. Walk on Rhode Island to 16th St. Right on 16th St.

18. Continue past San Francisco Center for the Book to De Haro.

19. Right on De Haro past St. Gregory of Nyssa Episcopal Church at No. 500.

20. Continue on De Haro to 19th St.

21. Left on 19th St. to Carolina.

22. Right on Carolina. Ascend stairway to 20th St.

23. Right on 20th St. to De Haro.

24. Left on De Haro to your beginning.

WALK 22 DESCRIPTION

◢ The walk begins in front of the Potrero Hill Neighborhood House (commonly called NABE, pronounced with a long *a*) at 953 De Haro at Southern Heights. It was founded in 1907 by the Presbyterian Church Women's Group to help immigrant groups learn English and cope with changes in their everyday lives. Since 1922, it has been located in architect Julia Morgan's Craftsman-style landmark building (No. 86).

◢ NABE continues in the spirit of Jane Addams's Hull House in Chicago and Neighborhood House in St. Paul (Adah's second home while she was growing up) in its relationship to the community. In addition to the array of activities available, including Head Start classes, senior lunches and socializing, and art and drama classes for young people, NABE is everybody's wonderful grandfather, an understanding listener, a protective and caring mentor. The legendary Enola Maxwell was the director of NABE from 1972 until her death in 2004. Her grandson, Edward Hatter, is the current director. The *Potrero View,* the community newspaper edited by volunteer Ruth Passen for 37 years, rents office space in the building. Steven Moss is the current publisher and editor.

◢ NABE is both the beginning of and the pivotal point in your walk. From here you have a continuous view in every direction. Orient yourself before proceeding: To the north, you have a close-up view of the downtown skyline; east, the Bay Bridge and Yerba Buena Island; south, Candlestick Hill; southwest, San Francisco General Hospital; and west, Twin Peaks.

◢ From NABE on De Haro, walk southeast along Southern Heights, curving left to 22nd St., at the crest of the hill. Among the foliage in the area is a Norfolk Island pine. Turning left on 22nd St., you pass a water reservoir built on an arresting serpentine rock formation. Descend the 22nd St. Stairway to Arkansas. This stairway is a pleasure to traverse because its proportion of riser to tread is exquisite. To the left of the stairway is a rocky area. Fennel grows well here, but it's impossible to use this area for a garden. At the bottom of the stairway, we are on Arkansas, which is not only pleasing to the eye but feels conducive to being a neighbor. Along this street and neighboring streets, there are a variety of trees from magnolia to ficus and passionflower vines.

⊿ Cross the street, and turn slightly to the right where you descend a wood plank stairway adjacent to the Connecticut Friendship Garden. In this area is a buckeye tree and coyote brush. Continue on the dirt path to Connecticut. The gate is on Connecticut, and if someone is working there, you may be able to enter. The small annual flower garden to the left of the poles may be an extension of the garden. To the right is the Potrero Hill Recreation Center.

⊿ Turn left on Connecticut. The architectural and botanical mix includes several Stick-style homes built in the 1880s (Nos. 524–512) and a variety of street trees, such as jacaranda, ficus, and Victorian box.

⊿ Turn left on 20th St. The Potrero Branch Library across the street at 1616 20th St. has a neighborhood archive collection, popular reading programs for children, and lectures for adults.

⊿ At Wisconsin you will see palms, ferns, and fuchsia. Continue to Carolina, and turn left. Walk on the right side of the street in order to better view the large serpentine outcropping upon which structures have been built. When you're almost opposite the Molokan Christian Church, walk up the stairway.

⊿ When you reach Southern Heights, turn right, as it curves to Rhode Island. Turn left on Rhode Island. As you walk downhill, you will notice a cottage, known as a "tuck-in," situated near the back of the lots on the right. This particular one was built around 1910. On the left, houses are built high on the hill. Next to No. 949, you can see the radio antennae on San Bruno Mountain. Bernal Heights, with its antiquated microwave station, is on the rise to the right of the mountain. Silhouettes of the hills are clearly delineated.

⊿ Turn right on 22nd St. Go down the short, steep 22nd St. (sidewalk) Stairway. Pass Kansas, and bear right on Vermont. On the slope to your right, agave, morning glory, and cypress trees are growing. A sound wall on the left mitigates some of the heavy traffic noise of US Highway 101.

⊿ Walk up Vermont, and ascend the stairway on the right in front of the houses into McKinley Square Park.

William Wordsworth walked 14 miles a day in his beloved English Lake District, and an estimated 185,000 miles in his lifetime.

⬕ Curve around the walkway to the left. You will see swirls of steam from the San Francisco General Hospital laundry facility. People come here to enjoy the park and rejuvenate. One time Adah met a gentleman reading contentedly at the redwood table under the cypress, and dogs and their owners often use the nearby designated dog run. Renovated and redesigned by landscape architect John Thomas, the park was dedicated in September 1999. When the mayor gave the signal, a group of neighborhood children snipped the official ribbon. The new playground is colorful and attractive to children who enjoy exploring the various shapes of play equipment. New benches are very convenient for picnicking and enjoying views; they give youngsters a great opportunity to identify city landmarks.

⬕ Beyond the play area, you descend the short stairway to the corner of San Bruno and 20th St. Here on top of the low retaining wall along the sidewalk is a brass US Geodetic Survey reference mark, which was placed here in 1932. At San Bruno and 20th St., cross the street, and walk along San Bruno to look at the flourishing Potrero Hill Community Garden.

⬕ Continue on San Bruno. Sunbursts adorn the three gables on Nos. 713–715. The block has flat-front Italianates, many of them redone with "misguided improvements," as architectural historian Judith Lynch so aptly described them. A shingled building, No. 636, has pleached ficus street trees in front and around the corner. No. 619, built in 1913, and No. 609, built in 1910, are some of the older homes in this section. A mini park, the Benches, is located at 18th St. You also have a view of Twin Peaks from here. (A skywalk extends across US Highway 101.)

⬕ Turn right on 18th St. and left on Vermont. The Slovenian Hall is at the left corner of Vermont at Mariposa. Turn right. The early Greek settlement was in this section. Light industry and small entrepreneurial firms are located in the lowlands north of Mariposa, to your left.

⬕ Continue on Mariposa toward Rhode Island. Turn left on Rhode Island to No. 350, built in 2002 on the site of a recycling center. To give a historic perspective, the architect used glass shards as part of the wall in the courtyard. Heavy metal grates hold back the glass. Turn right onto 16th St. A few feet from the corner is the San Francisco Center for the Book. One of the most active chapters in the country, they offer classes in various forms of the book arts, from traditional to experimental; there are classes in the use of the letterpress, and they teach children about bookmaking. You are welcome to come in

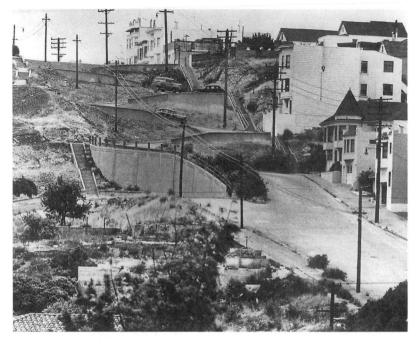

Potrero Hill, ca. 1950   *Courtesy of San Francisco Archives*

to see the exhibits Monday through Friday and attend public events. For more information, call 415-565-0545.

◢ Continue on 16th St. to De Haro, and turn right. Continue to 500 De Haro where you see St. Gregory of Nyssa Episcopal Church, which was built in 1995 and designed by architect John Goldman. St. Gregory parish places strong emphasis on liturgy that is grounded in Jewish and early-Christian practice. They believe in unconditional hospitality, a strong sense of community, and in music and dance, all of which is expressed in the shape of the entrance—a large, octagonal open space with an encircling mural depicting joyous dancing saints. After the liturgy in the adjoining room, the congregation reenters the open space and dances, reflecting the movements of the saints. A table is set with food for the congregation to partake.

◢ Across the street at 1705 Mariposa is the home of Anchor Brewing Company, one of the finest small breweries in the country. Its history goes back to the 1860s when it brewed one beer that was available only on tap. Now Anchor produces six handcrafted beers, plus a selection of seasonal beers. Tours are given twice each day, Monday–Friday by reservation only. Call 415-863-8350, extension 0 (Monday–Friday, 9 a.m.–4 p.m.), to make a reservation.

◢ Continue on De Haro toward 19th St. You pass Enola D. Maxwell Middle School of the Arts at No. 655, and soon after, an open space that contains remnants of a garden. You can see the Bay Bridge from here.

◢ Turn left on 19th St. to Carolina, and then right on Carolina to ascend the Carolina Stairway to 20th St. At the top are redwoods. The right-of-way has evolved into a garden with trees, agave, ivy, and shrubs. The Victoria Mews Association maintains the garden.

◢ Turn right on 20th St. to De Haro. A large embankment of serpentine rock at the southwest corner is the location of Francisco de Haro's adobe cottage built here in the 1830s. He was chosen as the first Mexican *alcalde* (Spanish for "mayor") of Yerba Buena in 1834.

◢ Turn left on De Haro, and walk on the left side in order to have a better view of the new architecture on the right. Continue on De Haro. Across the street from NABE, a mini park is being constructed, where a memorial plaque honors neighborhood activist Ruth Davidow. Cross the street to your beginning.

Further Rambling

From Potrero Hill, you can follow the old line of the ridge that ran to the Bay (since quarried away for landfill). Take 20th east from the end of Walk 22, passing the state streets as you go, eventually arriving at an overpass to US Highway 101. A few more blocks east, you can connect Walk 22 with Walk 31 in Dogpatch, at 18th and Mariposa. And if you trek east, visit Esprit Park at 20th and Indiana, where lovely redwoods and native plants along gravel trails are waiting quietly for you. This further ramble is mostly flat, but the emerging view from the overpass down to the water is compelling.

ʃtairway Trails

Bernal Heights East

The streets of Bernal Heights East meet at angles that vary from the rectangular grid. Also, street names can flip-flop within a block, and several streets converge at a "corner." Adah has mentioned these facts to several residents, who did seem surprised, but they understand the system.

Bernal Heights sits high above a maze of major thoroughfares—Alemany, Mission, and Cesar Chavez Streets, US Highway 101, and Interstate 280. It is part of what was once the Rancho de las Salinas y Potrero Nuevo (the Salinas ranch and pasture), granted to Jose Cornelio de Bernal in 1839 by the Mexican government. In the 1860s, the rancho (one league square, approximately 4,000 acres) was subdivided, and Vitus Wackenreuder made a survey of Bernal Heights. Wackenreuder plotted his streets narrow and his lots small—23 by 76 feet. Most of them do not meet today's city minimum size specifications. The east slope exceeds a 45% grade in many places, and its geological composition has hazardous landslide potential.

After the area was subdivided, the first settlers were predominantly Irish. They farmed the land and engaged in dairy ranching, the first extensive industry in Bernal Heights. Wakes were the most popular social gatherings, along with the telling of stories by "them as had the gift." The day Widow O'Brien's best milk cow was taken to the city pound and all her neighbors helped her get it back provided a true neighborhood story, endlessly told.

German and Italian settlers followed the Irish to Bernal Heights. During World War II, there was an influx of people, mainly blue-collar, from all over the United States, who came to work in the nearby naval shipyards. More recently, white-collar professionals have been moving into the neighborhood, attracted by the sunny climate and the neighborhood ambiance of the village within the city. Since 1995, the east slope of Bernal Heights has experienced fundamental and dramatic changes. A capital improvement project from sales tax monies has brought the streets into compliance with mandated safety codes. Along with improved streets

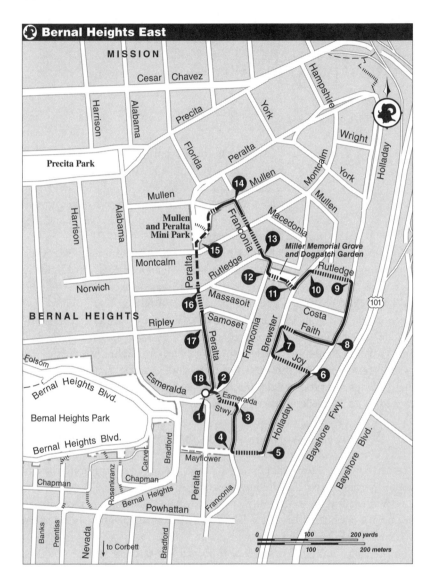

and water lines, the area now has, as of this latest writing, 50-plus stairways, with many of them constructed in the unused rights-of-way and on hills too steep to construct a street. The east slope is now one grand forest of stairway trails to explore.

QUICK-STEP INSTRUCTIONS

1. Begin at the corner of Peralta 600 and Esmeralda 1000.

2. Veer right to descend the unmarked Esmeralda Stairway.

3. Right on the 400 block of lower Franconia; continue to the right.

4. Left to descend the unmarked Mayflower Stairway.

5. Left on Holladay to Joy Stairway.

6. Left to ascend Joy Stairway to Brewster.

7. Right on Brewster to Faith Stairway, and descend.

8. Continue to Holladay, and turn left.

9. Ascend Rutledge Stairway next to No. 300 Holladay, and continue beyond the Mullen cul-de-sac to Brewster.

10. Left on Brewster to end of the retaining wall.

11. Bear right up the stairway. At first landing, turn left. Ascend stairway through community garden to Franconia.

12. Right on Franconia to Rutledge. Turn left.

13. Descend Franconia Stairway. Cross Montcalm, and continue to Mullen.

14. Left on Mullen. Ascend the stairway ramp to the open-space area. Follow path to Montcalm and Peralta.

15. Cross Montcalm, and continue up Peralta walkway. Ascend short stairway to Rutledge.

16. Cross Rutledge to ascend Peralta Stairway.

17. Continue on Peralta past Ripley.

18. Right on Esmeralda to your beginning.

WALK FACTS

Every Labor Day, the Bernal Heights Outdoor Cinema group hosts an annual festival that showcases films, videos, and live music with locals and filmmakers alike around the hill. They also present quarterly indoor screenings in conjunction with the Bernal Heights Branch Library and other venues and offer scholarships to young filmmakers.

The Illegal Soap Box Derby is held annually in Bernal Heights, though it sometimes gets shut down.

Early risers may want to visit the Alemany Flea Market; come early to find the best deals. It is open on Sundays, 8 a.m.–3 p.m., at 100 Alemany Blvd., the intersection of US Highway 101 and Interstate 280.

Walks 23 and 24 both have stairways named Esmeralda.

Bus Routes & Parking

PUBLIC TRANSPORTATION: MUNI Bus #67 Bernal Heights. For MUNI bus information, call 311 (outside San Francisco, call 415-701-2311).

PARKING: There is metered street parking available; metered parking is usually available for up to an hour, and free street parking is usually allowed for up to two hours. But also look for street-cleaning times posted in the neighborhood to avoid getting ticketed or towed.

WALK 23 DESCRIPTION

⬛ Begin at the "corner" of Peralta 600 and Esmeralda 1000. Across the street is the unmarked Esmeralda Stairway, which you descend to Franconia. Lovely landscaping and improved amenities set the tone for an adventure along the improved Bernal Heights stairways. You'll see plum trees, pines, and various annuals. A provided platform enables you to sit on a bench and look toward Hunters Point and the East Bay hills.

⬛ Turn right on the 400 block of Franconia. Several redwood-shingled houses dominate the street. Next to No. 447, turn left onto the unmarked Mayflower Stairway to Holladay. Two palm trees have been planted at the beginning of the descent. At the next to last landing, you have a view of India Basin and Oakland.

⬛ Continue down through the driveway to Holladay, and turn left. The traffic noise from the Bayshore Freeway (US Highway 101) is mitigated by double-paned windows and other insulation installed in the new and remodeled homes along the street. The slope is privately owned and consists of 13 lots. Some efforts to build were stalled by the neighbors who are hoping to keep it as open space.

⬛ Turn left at Joy Stairway, where a corkscrew willow tree has been planted. The first Joy Stairway was made up of a few steps that led up to a pulpitlike structure and then continued in a haphazard fashion up to Brewster. The slope was slippery and muddy then because of the heavy rains of 1982–83. The ambiance was rural with gingham and calico accents. More than two decades later, the new pedestrian thoroughfares were built to conform to safety codes. And yet another decade later, the area remains pleasant and walkable. Even with all these past improvements, the past holds on quite well. No. 18 Joy is an original flat-front Italianate from the 1870s.

⬚ Continue up the wood stairway to Brewster. Across from No. 138 Brewster, turn right and descend Faith Stairway. This concrete stairway traverses a garden of sweet peas, poppies, lavender, *Ceanothus*, coast live oaks, and pines. At the top, on the right, No. 159 Faith, built in 1901, features a stained-glass window. No. 137 Faith was connected to water in 1934, and No. 132 Faith, in 1944. From here, the skywalk that arches over the Bayshore Freeway looks attractive.

Will Kemp, the Shakespearean clown, jigged the 100 miles from London to Norwich on a bet in February 1600.

⬚ From the bottom of the stairs, continue to Holladay. Turn left on Holladay, and walk past Costa to Rutledge Stairway (next to No. 300 Holladay). It is an unmarked street right-of-way. You ascend the timber and metal stairway through a garden of redwoods, pines, a buckeye tree, and annuals. Walk up the concrete stairs. At the top is the cul-de-sac of Mullen.

⬚ To the right, the city land is planted with trees. To the left, the stairway continues where you ascend past some cottages. No. 43 Rutledge, built in 1895, is especially attractive in its setting among garden vines and trees on the lot. No. 55 Rutledge, on the left-side corner at Brewster, has an old-fashioned porch along the front of the house and some sculptures in the front garden.

⬚ Continue left on Brewster, walk past the retaining wall, and then turn right immediately to ascend the stairway. The Miller Memorial Grove and Dogpatch Garden is on your right. Bear left and ascend the stairway through the Community Garden. At the top, pass through the gate with the sign "This is a nice neighborhood garden."

⬚ You are now on Franconia. Turn right and then left on Rutledge to descend the stairway to Montcalm. The slope with the newly designed stairway and garden plots is the result of cooperation by neighbors.

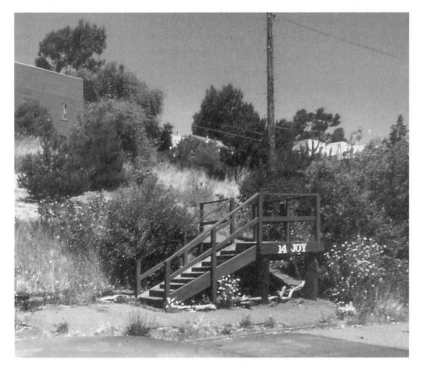

This historical photograph shows the Joy Stairway in 1983.   *Adah Bakalinsky*

The project sped along at an amazing rate (one year) due to good planning, excellent collaboration with the Department of Public Works and the Division of Street-Use Permits and some serendipities: One of the neighbors, an architect, facilitated the acquisition of permits by promptly completing the technical drawings required by the city; one of the neighbors is a contractor who donated his employees' labor to build the stairway; and another neighbor assisted with fundraising and publicity; and San Francisco Beautiful contributed. The ribbon cutting was Sunday, November 14, 2004.

◢ Cross Montcalm, and continue to Mullen. No. 109 Franconia is a Craftsman-style home that has an award-winning garden along Montcalm. Turn left on Mullen. Continue on the left side to ascend the stairway ramp. You pass a Japanese-style compound of several residences, built around a common courtyard.

◢ Follow the path to the crest of Peralta Point. City street rights-of-way and open-space funding contributed to this open area's establishment; it provides views of the downtown skyline from the Rincon towers to Twin Peaks. Plans for restoring native plants are in place.

◢ Continue left on the pathway adjacent to the open-space garden around the point, and walk ahead to Montcalm. Veer right, and cross Montcalm. Turn left on Peralta, and follow the walkway and short stairway, composed of different-sized and -colored steps.

◢ Cross Rutledge, and ascend the Peralta Stairway. At the top, you get a view of San Francisco that may make you catch your breath. The house on your right has an unusual fan-shaped fence. A redwood tree is at the corner of Samoset and Peralta. Continue on Peralta, past Ripley to Esmeralda and your beginning.

Further Rambling

If you feel hardy, or if it's time to enjoy that picnic you've been carrying around with you, hike up to Bernal Heights Park. From Esmeralda, walk up to Bradford St., then cross Bernal Heights Blvd. into Bernal Heights Park. This park allows dogs off-leash and also provides parking.

Circling Two Hills

Bernal Heights West

Sunny Bernal Heights enjoys extraordinary views of the city. With the largest number of stairways of any neighborhood, it also has a greater variety of street names with historic associations than any other. Among them you find: Banks, Winslow, Putnam, Army, Moultrie, and Sumter that relate to the Civil War; Powhattan, Samoset, and Massasoit that relate to Native American leaders; and several that relate to the US Colonial period. Bernal Heights has streets that change names, corners that don't coincide, some unpaved paths, and some of the most dedicated and active neighborhood-watch groups in the city. Neighbors here know how to work and cooperate with city agencies; they have been successful in establishing and preserving open space and community gardens wherever feasible.

WALK FACTS

Bernal Heights hosts an annual street fair, called Fiesta on the Hill, which includes petting zoos, dancing, two stages of live music, and pony rides. Proceeds benefit the Bernal Heights Neighborhood Center; call 415-206-2140 for details.

The Bernal Heights Farmers' Market, the longest-running farmers' market in the city, has been operating every Saturday since 1947.

If you like garage sales, come to the Bernal Heights Hill-wide Garage Sale held every August, where people in the neighborhood sell things they no longer need. Contact the Bernal Heights Neighborhood Center for more information and a map.

Walks 23 and 24 both have stairways named Esmeralda.

Bus Routes & Parking

PUBLIC TRANSPORTATION: MUNI Bus #24 Divisadero. For MUNI bus or Metro information, call 311 (outside San Francisco, call 415-701-2311).

PARKING: There is metered street parking available; metered parking is usually available for up to an hour, and free street parking is usually allowed for up to two hours. But also look for street-cleaning times posted in the neighborhood to avoid getting ticketed or towed.

WALK 24 DESCRIPTION

⊿ Begin your walk in an unusual circular configuration at Holly Park. Real estate developers gave it to the city in the 1860s hoping that an elite neighborhood would develop here, as it did in South Park, but the neighborhood became working class around 1900.

⊿ Ascend the concrete stairway at Holly Park Circle and Bocana. Follow the circular path clockwise around the park. Rockrose, marguerites, *Salvia,* irises, and boxwood bushes have been planted along the slopes. Holly Hill (274 feet) provides a view around the cardinal points of the compass. Behind you at the Bocana intersection is Bernal Heights Hill (325 feet), your destination. You can also see the dark, carnelian granite Bank of America Building in the Financial District.

⊿ Follow the walkway, and at Newman, look for the grove of olive trees transplanted from the Civic Center in 1998 that lines this eastern section of Holly Hill, as does a grove of eucalyptus. Near the Park St. intersection, you can see the Bayview District and Hunters Point. Looking south from the Murray intersection, you can see the blue water tower in McLaren Park. Continue on the path that dips down to the Appleton intersection, from where you see the buildings of Diamond Heights.

⊿ Cross Holly Park Circle at Appleton, and turn right to Elsie. You pass the College Hill Reservoir, built in the mid–19th century to bring water to the Mission District. Along the sidewalk, you also pass Elsie Garden, the work of talented and caring neighbors. At No. 324 Elsie is a jacaranda tree. Turn left at Santa Marina, and turn right next to No. 101 to descend the Prospect Stairway to Cortland. Walk through the Good Prospect Community Garden. It has a great variety of plants: roses, sweet peas, thyme, lemon verbena, Russian sage, vegetables, and fruit trees.

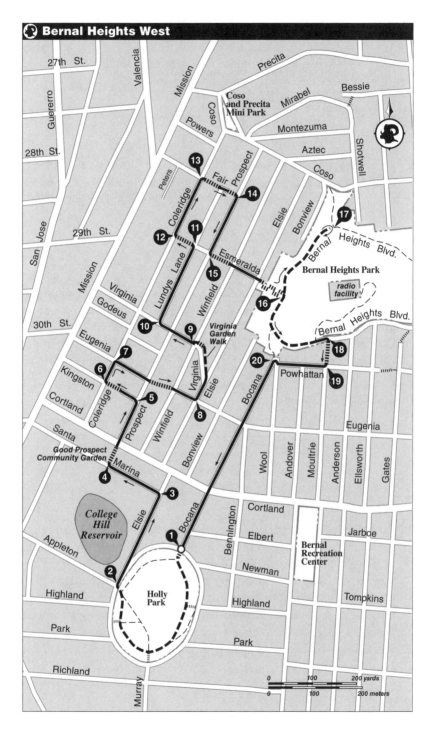

QUICK-STEP INSTRUCTIONS

1. Begin at Holly Park Circle and Bocana. Ascend stairway into Holly Park. Walk clockwise on circular path to Appleton and Elsie.

2. Cross Holly Park Circle, turn right, and walk to Elsie.

3. Continue on Elsie to Santa Marina. Turn left.

4. Right to descend Prospect Stairway to Kingston.

5. Left to Kingston Stairway to Coleridge.

6. Right on Coleridge to Eugenia.

7. Right on Eugenia. At Prospect ascend Eugenia Stairway to Winfield. Continue to intersection of Virginia and Elsie.

8. Cross the street to No. 199 Elsie. Left of where the two roads merge (the gore point), cross to No. 319 Virginia.

9. Walk to the end of Virginia Garden Walk. Descend short stairway. Continue past Winfield and Prospect to Lundys Lane.

10. Right on Lundys Lane to Esmeralda.

11. Left to descend Esmeralda Stairway.

12. Right on Coleridge to Fair.

13. Right to ascend Fair Stairway to Prospect.

14. Right on Prospect to Esmeralda.

15. Left to ascend Esmeralda Stairway to Bernal Heights Blvd.

16. Left on Bernal Heights Blvd. for views.

17. Return on Bernal Heights Blvd., past Esmeralda, to Moultrie.

18. Right to descend Moultrie Stairway to Powhattan.

19. Right on Powhattan to Bocana.

20. Left on Bocana to your beginning.

◢ Continue on Prospect, and turn left on Kingston. Follow the walkway to the concrete and steel stairway, built alongside the Franciscan Formation. You can see the nonidentical twin spires of St. Paul's Church in Noe Valley, and above it, Diamond Heights and Twin Peaks. Turn right on Coleridge to Eugenia. Walk uphill to the angled Eugenia Stairway, which is indicated by bollard posts, has a eucalyptus tree, and is flanked by agave and ivy and shaded by gingko and pine trees. A sign announces, "Eugenia Garden."

◢ At the top you cross Winfield, continue on Eugenia, and turn left at the combination Virginia and Elsie. The street then divides—Virginia

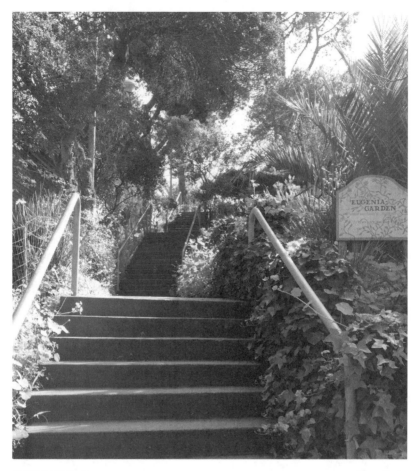

Eugenia Stairway   *Mary Burk*

goes downhill and Elsie up. Cross the street to No. 199 Elsie. Turn left and walk to the uphill side of the gore point, where you see two roads merging, just past the one-way sign; cross the street there. Walk on the sidewalk to the left of No. 319, the shingled house with tile accents. Follow the Virginia Garden Walk, another neighborhood beautification project.

⌁ Go past the two stairways to your left, follow the left curve, and descend the third stairway. The sign "Virginia Garden Walk" is to the left. Cross Winfield. No. 217 Virginia is a three-story Stick-style Italianate. Continue down mostly elm tree–lined Virginia.

- Pass Prospect, and turn right on Lundys Lane, one of Adah's favorite streets. Carob trees planted along the street complement the cottages here.

- Turn left to descend the concrete Esmeralda Stairway, which is enhanced by plantings of *Ceanothus,* sage, and daisies. At the top and bottom of the stairway are viewing platforms.

- Turn right on Coleridge. There is a Mini Park across the street. Continue to Fair; turn right and ascend the Fair Stairway. In 1990, a Cinco de Mayo celebration with costumed dancers and live music was performed at the top of the stairway. Continue past the brick-paved cul-de-sac of Lundys Lane.

- Turn right on Prospect, next to a garden with pines, eucalyptus, *Echium, Pelargonium,* and *Agapanthus.* Continue over the hill past No. 34, one of the oldest homes in Bernal Heights. Situated on the original goat farm, the homestead has been extended from a simple, narrow clapboard with gables to a roomy, two-story, eight-room structure.

  In 1885 Charles Lummis walked 3,500 miles, from Cincinnati, Ohio, to Los Angeles in 143 days. He paid for his trip by writing articles about his adventures for the Los Angeles Times. *He fought off a wildcat and a mountain lion, escaped from convicts, and set his own broken arm. Subsequently he became city editor of the newspaper.*

- Turn left onto another section of the Esmeralda Stairway—this one with steel handrails and lights, flowers along the edges, and rope swings hanging from the branches of tall trees. At the top of the stairway is the recently refurbished double slide. Adults like to try it, and they quickly arrive at the bottom. Several trees, including a large pepper, shade the picnic table and bench at the Winfield Plaza.

- Continue up the short block of Esmeralda to the highest section of the stairway. This section leads through a shade garden of ferns and rhododendrons, another project of caring neighbors. A stone monument is marked with a memorial plaque for the late Margaret Randolph, a Bernal Heights activist.

- At the top, surrounded by flowering plum and *Ceanothus,* is the asphalt road that circles Bernal Heights Park. Neighbors succeeded in having the city close this section of road to cars, making it safe for walkers. Designated as a "natural area," the hill is where the Bernal

Hilltop Native Grassland Restoration Project hosts work parties, on every third Saturday of the month, with volunteer opportunities scheduled through 2014. Contact the San Francisco Recreation and Parks Department (415-831-2700) for more information.

⌐ Many people jog or walk the 1-mile route around the hill too. The view from here is also one of the most rewarding in the city. Walk left as far as you like for the views, and then retrace your steps (south) to a west-facing bench where you can take in San Bruno Mountain, Twin Peaks, and Angel Island.

Esmeralda Stairway *Mary Burk*

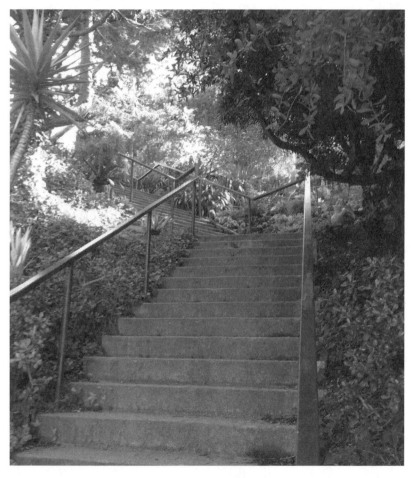

▄ Walk past Esmeralda, and continue on the road as it curves left past the auto barrier. Then walk to the end of the chain-link fence, and look for the beginning of the Moultrie Stairway, near the driveway of No. 123 (written on the wood fence), beside the multiple mailboxes. Bear right at the fence and left under a eucalyptus. The pebble-covered path with wood water-stop steps becomes concrete and goes past gardens. Walk on a ramp to Powhattan.

▄ Turn right and proceed along Powhattan to its end. The triangle-shaped garden across the street is a neighbor-initiated project.

▄ Turn left on Bocana to go downhill toward Holly Park and your beginning.

Further Rambling

Cortland, which you cross on the way to start or end Walk 24, is one of the major east–west streets in this neighborhood, and a lovely shopping street district with coffeehouses and restaurants worthy of repeat visits. The area happily attracts top chefs and restaurateurs ready to offer locals new things to amuse the palette.

Follow the Curve, Follow the View

Diamond Heights, Fairmount Heights & Glen Canyon Park

The Diamond Heights neighborhood was built on 325 acres of craggy, hilly terrain after World War II, when federal redevelopment money became available for construction. A range of modest to luxurious homes, town houses, apartments, and condominiums were built, trees were planted, and stairways were constructed. Diamond Heights is bounded by important corridor streets, including O'Shaughnessy, Portola, Clipper, and Diamond Heights Blvd., and by the 300-foot-deep Glen Canyon Park, which separates it from Miraloma to the west and Glen Park to the east.

WALK FACTS

Glen Canyon is especially gorgeous and quiet in the morning after a rainstorm.

Nonnative trees felled in 2013 have not been replaced, nor have any other noise-dampening measures been taken, making freeway noise nearby somewhat more apparent. Even though neighbors protested the change, more than 300 trees were removed.

During periods of heavy rain or restoration work, you cannot walk along the left side of Islais Creek. However, from the main road (the right side), you can see the plants that grow so well near and in water—willows, sedges, and *Equisetum* (horsetail). Native wild-flowers—sticky monkeyflower, coyote brush, red flowering currant, and columbine—grow on the slopes.

By walking across the wooden bridge past the north trail, you can see many birds, walkers, and their dogs and get a close look at the 300-foot canyon, which exposes a massive Franciscan Formation, rock found throughout San Francisco and in limited quantities elsewhere along the California coast.

Bus Routes & Parking

PUBLIC TRANSPORTATION: MUNI Bus #35 Eureka and #52 Excelsior. The Glen Park BART station is in the area. For MUNI bus information, call 311 (outside San Francisco, call 415-701-2311).

PARKING: There is street parking, which is usually allowed for 2 hours, but also look for street-cleaning times posted in the neighborhood to avoid getting ticketed or towed.

WALK 25 DESCRIPTION

⊿ Beginning at the shopping-center corner of Diamond Heights Blvd. (No. 5290) and Gold Mine, walk right up Diamond Heights Blvd. At the next intersection, turn left on Diamond, and follow the curve to Beacon. It's a great place to take visitors for the remarkable vista. Walk along the ridge of Beacon on the sidewalk to No. 425, then cross the street to a footpath. Here we see cycle tracks and footpaths crisscrossing the slope of Billy Goat Hill. Bernal Heights Park and its radio tower are visible straight ahead on the hill.

⊿ The Harry Stairway begins between Nos. 190 and 200 Beacon. It is very easy to miss because it looks like a private walkway. The stairway is constructed of both wood and concrete. You descend parallel to numerous conifers growing in the lot on the right. Monterey cypress branches overhang the stairway. An urban street and a forest path have a surprisingly pleasing contrast in atmosphere and vegetation, and from the long Harry Stairway you can see the variety in homes alongside it, which establishes an individual style for the vicinity.

⊿ When you're on the lower concrete steps, you can see Yerba Buena Island and the Bay Bridge to the east and the spires of St. Paul's Church and downtown San Francisco to the north. All the while, closer to you, African daisies, ivy, geraniums, wild onions, *Pittosporum,* yuccas, lilies of the Nile, daturas, *Abutilon,* nasturtium, and hydrangeas provide a celebration of color and foliage.

⊿ The Harry Stairway ends at Laidley No. 100. You are now in the Fairmount Heights neighborhood, which was platted in 1864. The boundaries are Castro to the west, Arlington to the east, 30th St. to the north, and Bemis to the south. Cobb and Sinton were the real estate

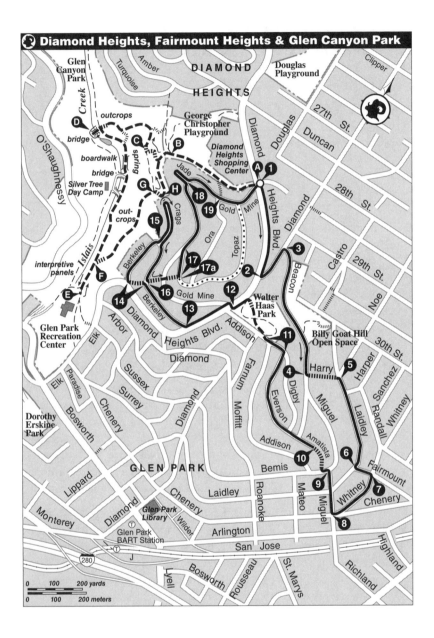

Diamond Heights, Fairmount Heights & Glen Canyon Park

QUICK-STEP INSTRUCTIONS

1. From Diamond Heights Blvd. shopping center (No. 5290) and Gold Mine, walk south on Diamond Heights Blvd. to Diamond St.

2. Left on Diamond St. to Beacon.

3. Right on Beacon to Harry Stwy., next to No. 190 Beacon.

4. Descend stairway to Laidley.

5. Right on Laidley.

6. Left on Fairmount.

7. Right on Whitney.

8. Right to Chenery, and right again on Miguel.

9. Left on Bemis, and then right to ascend Amatista Stairway to Everson.

10. Bear left on Everson. Continue to end of street at "Digby 000" sign.

11. Turn left on Digby, and cross Addison. Right into Haas Park, and left to ascend stairway to Diamond Heights Blvd.

12. Cross Diamond Heights Blvd. Left on it to Berkeley Way.

13. Right on Berkeley Way.

14. Next to No. 101, left to descend Onique Stairway. Right on Berkeley Way, and cross street to see canyon and rock formations near the corner of Crags Ct. Bear right.

15. Now turn left. Go to end of Crags Ct. Return to Berkeley Way. Bear left.

16. Next to No. 100 Berkeley Way, ascend Onique Stairway to No. 400 Gold Mine. Continue up stairway to No. 243 Topaz.

17. Left on Topaz. Right on Gold Mine.

17a. *Optional but lovely:* Right on Topaz. Right on Gold Mine to your beginning.

18. Walk into Jade Place, and return to Gold Mine.

19. Continue on Gold Mine to Diamond Heights Blvd. and your beginning.

developers. Old photos show vernacular cottages along unpaved paths and pine groves.

⬛ Turn right on Laidley. A short street (one of Adah's favorites), it is, essentially, a street of cottages. A resident of the street, Architect Jeremy Kotas has been responsible for the dramatic metamorphosis from simple cottages to imaginative, contemporary dwellings. You pass several homes he worked on: Nos. 102, 123, 128, 134, 135, and 140. No. 134 is known as the Sand Castle because of its undulating first story, and No. 140 is known in the neighborhood as the Owl House because of its curving features that resemble eyebrows.

QUICK-STEP INSTRUCTIONS Glen Canyon

A. Walk in area from Diamond Heights Blvd. and Gold Mine Drive to George Christopher Playground along the path to the left.

B. Take the left path into the canyon, and descend first log-and-plank stairway.

C. Continue on paths and log and plank stairways toward the right. The path ends on the road near the bridge.

D. Left to cross bridge and boardwalk. Continue walking on either side of Islais Creek toward the Glen Park Recreation Center building.

E. The interpretive panel near the recreation center outlines the trails in the canyon: Christopher Park, Crags Court, and Berkeley Way.

F. To return, walk to the next interpretive panel by the light post. Ascend path with log and plank stairways, continuing along the outcrops toward Crags Court.

G. Continue on right path at junction, and ascend toward Crags Court.

H. Just before Crags Court, turn left on path back to your beginning.

"A walk should have simplicity and complexity, contrast and unity." —A. Packerman

The palatial three-story Second Empire and Italianate home, Nos. 192–196 (near Fairmount), now an apartment house, was built in 1872. It is commonly known as the Bell Mystery House. The death of the owner, Thomas Bell, a San Francisco financier, occurred under mysterious circumstances in 1892. His wife, Teresa, and his housekeeper, Mary Ann Pleasant, may have been involved. Without a satisfactory explanation, it has been fodder for a neighborhood myth. Pleasant (known as Mammy Pleasant) is the most interesting character in the story. A free-born black woman from Philadelphia, dedicated abolitionist, and entrepreneur, she was a celebrated cook who worked for wealthy families. She owned laundries, boardinghouses, and brothels. (For more information about her, see *Mammy Pleasant* and *Mammy Pleasant's Partner* both by Helen Holdredge and *A Cast of Hawks* by Milton Gould.)

Turn left on Fairmount. No. 226 is a tuck-in, set deep into the lot where residents can enjoy an enviable view. Make a right turn on Whitney, a small street with several row Queen Annes. Turn right to Chenery, the Glen Park neighborhood shopping street. Farther along the street, a coffeehouse, a bakery, the hardware store, and Bird & Beckett Books and Records convey the essence of a small town Main St. A new branch library was opened in February 2010 at 2825 Diamond.

- Turn right on Miguel, and walk uphill to Bemis. Turn left and then right to ascend the Amatista Stairway to Everson. A shopping center was proposed for the triangle near the top of the stairs, but residents opposed it, and the area is now a small park.

- Everson is one of the oldest sections of the Diamond Heights Redevelopment Area. A resident told me that her home and the house at No. 50 Everson, which was made with lumber from the 1939 Golden Gate International Exposition on Treasure Island, were the only two structures on the street in 1957.

- Continue on the left side of Everson for the view: Bayview Heights, the blue water tower of the Excelsior neighborhood, and San Bruno Mountain with its radio towers. Walk past the "Digby 100" street sign. Continue to the end of Everson at the "Digby 100" sign.

Harry Stairway   *Tony Holiday*

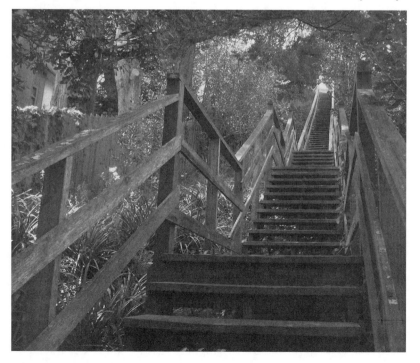

⊿ Turn left, pass the fire station, cross Addison, and walk right through the basketball court of the 4-plus-acre Walter Haas Park and Playground, an inviting place for picnicking, playing, and just sitting.

⊿ Walk up the short stairway to Diamond Heights Blvd. If you'd like to return to the beginning of the walk at this point, turn right. If you'd like to continue on to the Diamond Heights portion of the walk, cross the boulevard and turn left. You pass a sign that reads "Gold Mine 000 End." Continue on Diamond Heights Blvd. to Berkeley Way.

⊿ At Berkeley Way turn right. Next to No. 101, descend Onique Stairway to the lower loop of Berkeley Way. Turn right on Berkeley Way, and cross the street. You are looking down on Glen Canyon Park, where, in the 1800s, carnivals, parades, picnics, dances, and other amusements took place. Continue farther to see the extraordinary rock formation near the corner of Crags Court. One of the first residents on Crags bought a house here to practice rock climbing.

⊿ Veer right, and turn left at the corner. Continue to the end of Crags. A thriving community garden exists in this area. The people who attend

To Crags Court　　　　　　　　　　　　　　　　　　*Tony Holiday*

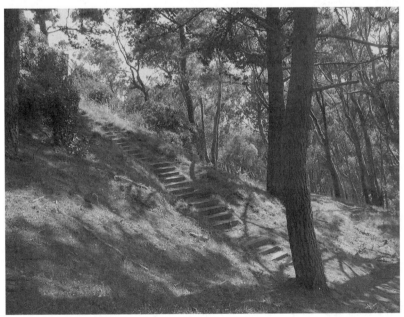

it welcome visitors and will share their knowledge and samples of fruits and flowers.

◢ Return to the upper loop of Berkeley Way. Eucalyptus and pine trees have been planted here and in the hills (right) above O'Shaughnessy. Walk on the left side. Next to No. 100 Berkeley Way, ascend Onique Stairway. Midway up it, you're next to No. 400 Gold Mine. Cross the street, and continue upward. At the top, we are next to No. 243 Topaz.

◢ Turn left on Topaz and right on Gold Mine (679 feet). Turn left into Jade Place for limited views of the Sutro Tower, Mt. Davidson, and San Bruno Mountain between the houses and garages. As you return to Gold Mine, you are confronted by the incongruous placement of the Rincon towers next to our iconic Bay Bridge, which Adah calls the Cinderella Bridge. It's a carrier of heavy traffic during the day and, in the evening, a graceful structure within the bridge lights. Continue around to your left, walking downhill on Gold Mine to the beginning.

◢ An optional, enjoyable route is to turn right on Topaz. As you walk along the ridge near No. 131, an extraordinary view unfolds before you—east and south. Continue down the hill to Gold Mine; bear right to your beginning.

◢ You may want to take the alternate route in Glen Canyon Park (Steps A–H on the map) upon your return to Diamond Heights Blvd., or perhaps you prefer to enjoy it at another time. Watch your step because the paths are narrow. You may want to use a walking stick.

Further Rambling

Chenery, the "downtown" Glen Park, has the atmosphere of a small town main street with its restaurants and stores. Visit the relatively new library at 2825 Diamond at Wilder. And try out the alternate walk (Steps A–H) sometime.

A Harmonious Walk

McLaren Park & Excelsior

McLaren Park, located in the southeast corner of San Francisco, is the city's second largest park (318 acres) and one of its least known. On this walk, you'll explore the seeps, ponds, and marshes of the park's well-tended northern edge. By traversing bridges and stairways, you'll segue into the surrounding neighborhood, which retains a relatively rustic ambiance. All these elements mingle harmoniously here.

The park is dedicated to John McLaren, who was the chief gardener of Golden Gate Park for 60 years. While the city began purchasing land for the park in the late 1920s, its designated area was not fully acquired until the 1970s because of short funding and dozens of farming inholdings. In 1987, a bond issue providing $2.4 million to implement the master plan for McLaren Park was passed. It provided for a felicitous park design with cypress and redwood groves, cattail marshes, and riparian areas where willow and horsetail grow.

WALK FACTS

McLaren Park Summer Stage holds several community events and schedules live music at the Jerry Garcia Amphitheater each year. In 2013 the Jerry Day event, named for the artist who was from the Excelsior District, drew many people to the park.

If you see one of the coyotes that live in the park, back away slowly. If you have a dog with you, keep him leashed and far away from coyotes; he would likely lose if they were to fight.

The Excelsior Action Group engages with residents and merchants in the area to sponsor or facilitate community activities year-round; they work with such city agencies as the Planning Department, Department of Public Works, and the San Francisco Public Library.

Bus Routes & Parking

PUBLIC TRANSPORTATION: MUNI Bus #52 Excelsior and #54 Felton. For MUNI bus information, call 311 (outside San Francisco, call 415-701-2311).

PARKING: There is metered street parking available; metered parking is usually available for up to an hour, and free street parking is usually allowed for up to two hours. But also look for street-cleaning times posted in the neighborhood to avoid getting ticketed or towed.

WALK 26 DESCRIPTION

◢ Begin in the 300 block of Gambier at Felton, and walk toward Burrows. The attached houses on your left date from the 1940s and 1950s, but the cottages on the right are from the early 1900s. They occupy two or three lots with room for extensive yards and outbuildings. Gravel driveways and well-tended gardens lend them a rural touch.

◢ Enter McLaren Park from Burrows and Gambier. A neighbor enjoying the view from his porch once said that the park across the street was rough pasture when he moved here in 1961 and that it still feels as if he lives in the country. Note the tiered planter and mosaic bollards that the Friends of McLaren Park installed recently at this entrance.

◢ Proceed straight on an asphalt walkway that soon begins to descend around the top of a large grassy bowl. Along the trail are eucalyptus and Monterey pine groves (remnants of farm-era wood lots). Follow the curve of the trail along the redwood grove and by young live oaks. Keep left along the path parallel to Shelley. You glimpse the Portola and Bayview neighborhoods and the East Bay hills.

◢ Where the path meets wide Shelley Drive, there's a round sandbox in the middle. Across the street (right) is a large group picnic area. Proceed left from the sandbox, keeping left along the path.

◢ The path enters a grove of alder and redwood and crosses a concrete bridge. The creek below flows from a natural spring, just ahead to your left. Look for the horsetails (*Equisetum*). To see where it flows, turn right at the corner of Harvard and Bacon, walk for one block,

(Continued on page 222)

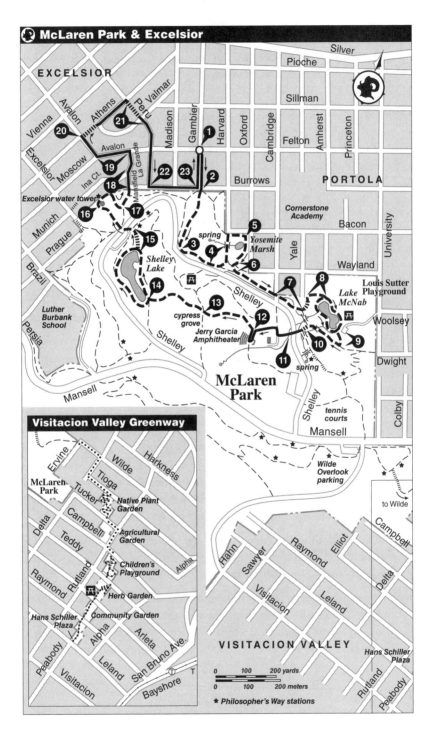

QUICK-STEP INSTRUCTIONS

1. Begin on 300 block of Gambier at Felton. Walk to Burrows.

2. Cross Burrows into McLaren Park. Continue straight on descending path.

3. Follow curve of trail along a eucalyptus grove and then a redwood grove.

4. Continue left from sandbox and across a concrete bridge.

5. Continue around left edge of Yosemite Marsh on asphalt path.

6. Right at basketball court; left to walk along path beside Shelley.

7. Cross Cambridge and continue on path; soon bear left and descend stairway to Yale.

8. Turn right down driveway to Lake McNab; circle either way around the lake.

9. Leave Lake McNab via sandy playground; ascend right on paved path.

10. After the footbridge, take left path up railroad-tie stairway. Then bear right on the side path to Shelley.

11. Cross Shelley and walk up opposite paved driveway. Bear right then left to handicap parking lot, to view amphitheater.

12. Return to parking lot gate. Bear left to go up the gravel path.

13. Where the path and trail intersect, bear left on gravel path; continue ahead at the cypress grove junction on the level path.

14. At the south tip of Shelley Lake, walk either way around the lake.

15. At the north end turn left. Climb long railroad-tie stairway to parking lot. Cross Shelley and ascend paved water tank driveway.

16. Circle counterclockwise around water tower to stone marker. Descend east via dirt path, keeping right at fork.

17. Turn left on paved path. Stay left at playground.

18. Exit park at corner of Burrows and Mansfield. Continue straight on Mansfield, which becomes La Grande, for one block.

19. Left on Avalon. Follow Avalon one block to Moscow, and right for another block to Athens.

20. Right and ascend Athens Stairway. Continue on Athens for one block to Peru.

21. Turn left up Peru Stairway to Valmar. Continue on Peru for two blocks to Burrows.

22. Left on Burrows to Gambier.

23. Left to 300 block of Gambier and your beginning.

(Continued from page 219)

and turn right again. On your right is a tiny pond filled with cattails. The water's surface is nearly covered with a floating carpet of duckweed. Though human-made, the pond is home to raccoons and small birds. It captures runoff from the grassy bowl you descended from Gambier and keeps the adjacent neighborhood dry.

◢ Continue around the left edge of the Yosemite Marsh on the asphalt path. Picnic tables, benches, a walkway, and plantings along the pond are some of the inviting aspects of this section. Beyond the round restroom, turn right at the basketball court, and clamber up a steep path to some large cypress trees.

"I love walking in London," said Mrs. Dalloway. "Really it's better than walking in the country." —Virginia Woolf, Mrs. Dalloway

◢ Now turn left and saunter along the path beside Shelley Drive, enjoying the broad views. Behind you is the pond; to your left is the Portola District. The tall, Italian-style tower is Cornerstone Academy, a private school occupying a former convent. To the east you can see the flat expanse of the University Mound Reservoir and get a glimpse of San Francisco Bay and the East Bay hills.

◢ At the intersection of Shelley and Cambridge, cross Cambridge, and descend a winding asphalt path through a dense pine grove. Bear left at the next two junctions. Railroad-tie steps descend to the end of Yale. Turn right and descend the paved driveway to Lake McNab, a human-made lake fed by natural springs and runoff from the north slope of McLaren Park. Two big cattail "islands" provide cover for many kinds of birds, including egrets, herons, ducks, and coots. Neighbors enjoy the stroll around the paved lakeshore. The California Conservation Corps helped to establish two islands for bird nesting and improve the habitat in this area. Work continues in the park, coordinated under the San Francisco Recreation and Parks Department.

◢ Walk either way around the lake to the far end, where you find a wood-topped drain cover, as well as some swings and a small sandbox in the Louis Sutter Playground; picnic tables provide a pleasant place to sit. Leaving the lake via the sandbox playground, ascend (right) along the paved path, leading past a thicket of willow and alder. Just beyond the first zigzag footbridge, take the left path with railroad-tie steps. Bear right on the short side path to wide Shelley Drive.

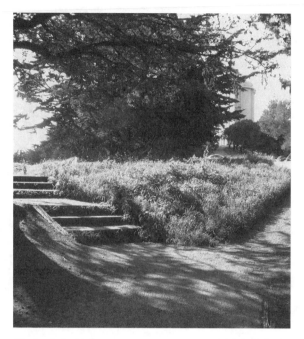

Shelley Lake Stairway   *Adah Bakalinsky*

◢ Cross Shelley carefully, and walk up the paved driveway opposite the Jerry Garcia Amphitheater. A farmhouse up ahead makes for a handy landmark; not quite rural, not quite urban, it's a remnant of the old greenhouses and farms that used to dot this area, as are the scattered palm trees down the valley. About 100 feet up the driveway, take the right fork. Turn left at the first opening, and follow the parking sign through the small lot for the handicapped. Ahead (left) is the stunning, renovated amphitheater. The Friends of the Jerry Garcia Amphitheater are working to increase the number and types of events held here, and the San Francisco Recreation and Parks Department's 2014 special events calendar already includes Jerry Day, the San Francisco Mountain Bike Festival, and Shakespeare in the Park.

◢ After viewing the amphitheater, return to the parking lot gate, and follow the gravel path to the left. As you climb, the path goes left through open grassland. Red-tailed hawks sometimes perch on the trees on the right of the path. At a cypress grove near the top of the hill is a complex intersection of paths and trails. Continue straight ahead on the level path, crossing a grassy slope edged with coyote

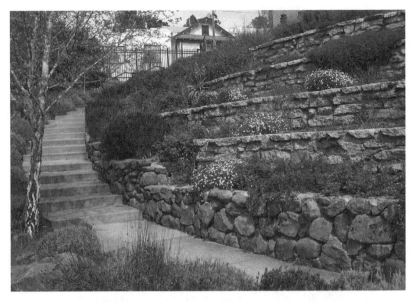

Visitacion Valley Greenway   *Annette Hovie*

brush. In the spring, native wildflowers are abundant (look, but don't pick!). Below (right) is the group picnic area you saw near the beginning of the walk.

◢ Your path leads to the south tip of Shelley Lake, a reservoir for the park's irrigation water. This lake is windier and more exposed than other sections of the park. A chain-link fence incompletely separates the lake (several openings let you get close to the water) from the rocky shoreline. Walk along either shore. At the north end, turn left and climb a long railroad-tie stairway to the crest of the hill.

◢ Continue past the parking lot to Shelley. The blue Excelsior water tower, a 50-year-old neighborhood landmark is on the hilltop ahead. The new tank was installed in 2007 and has the same water capacity—350,000 gallons. The water, which is from the Hetch Hetchy Reservoir in the Sierra Nevada, is for San Francisco's drinking water and fire protection. Cross Shelley, and ascend the long paved driveway. Circle counterclockwise around the water tower to enjoy the panoramic view, one of the grandest in the city. To the north are Bernal Heights, Diamond Heights, Glen Canyon, and Twin Peaks, plus a bit of the downtown skyline. To the west is City College, and to the south is the Excelsior District and San Bruno Mountain.

◢ When you are ready, retrace your steps toward Shelley, and turn left on the paved path. Stay left at the playground, and exit the park at the corner of Burrows and Mansfield. Take a look at No. 73 Mansfield, an unassuming little country house.

◢ Walk ahead one block on Mansfield, and then bear right on La Grande to Avalon. The church on the corner was formerly a neighborhood grocery store. Turn left on Avalon, and follow it (as it curves right) to Athens. Turn right, and ascend the concrete Athens Stairway. City College gradually comes into view. Continue on Athens for one block to Peru. Your view ahead is toward the northeast.

◢ Ascend Peru Stairway. The adjoining hillside was a dumping ground and an eyesore in the 1970s until a grassroots group, the Hilltop Block Club, banded together. In cooperation with the Recreation and Parks Department and the City's Open Space Committee, the club retained landscape architect Richard Schadt to design the hillside garden and stairway. Approximately 70 neighborhood residents cooperated in digging, planting, and watering more than 150 trees and shrubs, which had been propagated at the Golden Gate Park nursery. The basic work was completed in 1982.

◢ The serpentine stairway is built of aggregate and railroad ties. The trees on the slopes include Australian willow (*Myoporum*), Italian pine, and flowering plum. The view behind you includes Mt. Davidson (the one with the cross, which Walk 13 visits) and Glen Canyon Park (Walk 25).

◢ At the top you enter an open grassy knoll, Valmar Terrace (a perfect place to sit and read or simply gaze around). The neighbor on the left tends the area, watering, picking up garbage, and planting flowers on her adjoining lot so everyone can enjoy the greenery.

◢ Continue on Peru. (The view now takes in San Francisco General Hospital, the shipyards, Mt. Diablo across the Bay and to the left, Roundtop Peak.) No. 747 Peru is below street level. Lemon trees grow in the yard, and a penthouse faces east. To the right you see the blue water tower in McLaren Park again, and as you continue walking on Peru, you face the park.

◢ At Peru and Burrows, the uneven macadam road and adjoining McLaren Park can make you feel like you've been out for a country walk. Turn left on Burrows to reach Gambier and your beginning.

Further Rambling

Philosopher's Way is a 2.7-mile loop around McLaren Park's perimeter; you can access it from a couple points in this walk. At Step 15, near Shelley Lake, head north to find more markers on the main trail; the Yosemite Creek panel is the closest. At Step 10, walk up toward the spring, where there are more markers nearby. Philosopher's Way includes places to rest and view the landscape and also highlights the interconnected paths of the area's ecology, geography, and history, as well as the experiences of the people who come here. Walkers become part of the landscape, and their presence leaves traces—walk lightly. A copy of the trails included in Philosopher's Way is available at **savemclarenpark.org.**

Visitacion Valley Greenway is one of the finest examples of community work in San Francisco of neighborhood beautification, gardens, and parks. It is difficult not to return time after time to this 2-acre greenway developed from six publicly owned lots and extending over a six-block area. Each block has a specialized garden, sculptures, benches, and tiles. The project took 16 years; the first 5 were spent acquiring properties from the Public Utilities Commission, and the next 11 were spent building the structures and landscaping. In 2009 the last garden, an herb garden, was opened. Fran Martin and Anne Seeman were the prime movers. The decorative gates, fences, and tile work were created by Martin and sculptor Jim Growden.

The gardens begin on Leland Ave. across from Peabody St. at Hans Schiller Plaza in the business district. Then they wind through the neighborhood from Raymond to Tioga between Alpha and Delta from Community Garden to Herb Garden, Children's Playground, Agricultural Garden, and finally Native Plant Garden.

Views, Views, Views! A Hop from Hill to Hill

Four Hills

Adah has convinced me that a good walk takes on the shape of *something* real. Some of her walks even take on the fitting shape of a boot or a shoe. However, Adah's friend Charles Brock, who designed this walk, found a new shape—the Rabbit Hop. This lively walk encircles the Upper Market and the Twin Peaks areas. Do bring your binoculars. It's easy to forget that San Francisco has views all around its perimeter, not just from Telegraph Hill, Russian Hill, and Twin Peaks.

To walk in San Francisco is an adventure all its own. And this adventure takes walkers to Kite Hill, Tank Hill, Mount Olympus, and Corona Heights (Rock Hill). Monument Way, named for the statue it once hosted, is obscured by buildings crowded so close to the leftover monument pedestal that its former expansiveness has been lost. But, when Adolph Sutro presented the statue to the city in 1887, he offered this wish to the ceremonious crowd, "May the light shine from the torch of the Goddess of Liberty to inspire our citizens to good and noble deeds for the benefit of mankind." Sutro's triumphant gift to the city fell into disrepair and then was removed mysteriously from its pedestal sometime in 1955—never to be seen again. Knowing what was once there adds another dimension of mystery to your understanding of San Francisco.

Corona Heights, known as Rock Hill until 1941, is adorned with native plants, provides good areas for hiking, and offers great views of the Castro, Church, Market St., and downtown, all the way to the Ferry Building. Although reduced from its original size, this open space still invites you to come out and walk around.

(Continued on page 230)

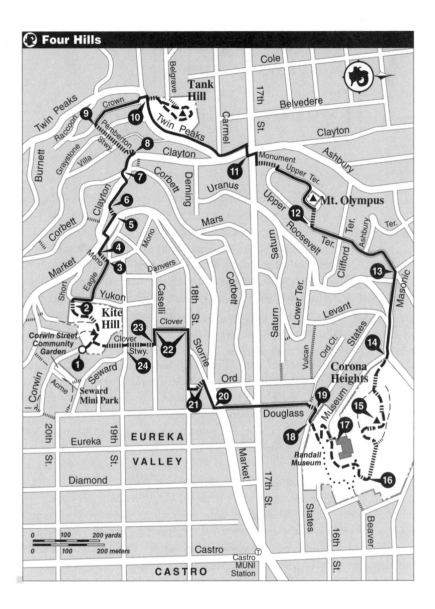

Four Hills

QUICK-STEP INSTRUCTIONS

1. From end of Corwin, enter Kite Hill Open Space, and follow trail to the left. Descend the stairway, and follow Yukon Trail ahead of you.
2. Right on Yukon, and then immediate left on Eagle.
3. Opposite No. 84 Eagle, ascend Mono Stairway to Market.
4. Right on Market, and walk up to the stoplight at Clayton. Cross Market at crosswalk.
5. Right on Market, proceed 250 feet, then left, and ascend the stairway to Clayton.
6. Right on Clayton to Corbett.
7. Cross Clayton and then Corbett, and walk up Clayton on the left side.
8. From the left side, ascend the Pemberton Stairway to Crown Terrace.
9. Right on Crown Terrace to Twin Peaks Blvd.
10. Cross Twin Peaks Blvd. at crosswalk, and ascend stairway to Tank Hill. Return to Twin Peaks Blvd., and then left to 17th St. and Clayton.
11. Right on 17th St., then immediately left to ascend the Monument Way Stairway. Bear left, then right around Mt. Olympus.
12. Next to No. 480, descend the stairway to Upper Terrace, and left to Masonic.
13. Right on Masonic, and then straight to Roosevelt and Museum Way.
14. Enter the gate at the fence. Stay right across the lawn, and ascend the stairway and trail above to the summit of Corona Heights.
15. Descend the stairway. Then left on the trail, and right to descend another, long stairway to the trail junction above the tennis courts.
16. Head straight for the back porch of the Randall Museum. Cross over the porch and around the museum (closed Sunday and Monday) to the parking lot.
17. Bear left and descend an asphalt path to States.
18. Right on States to No. 187, then left to descend stairway to Douglass.
19. Walk down Douglass, and cross Market at crosswalk.
20. Right on Market to Storrie.
21. Left to descend stairway to Ord and 18th St.
22. Right on 18th St. to Clover, then left on Clover to Caselli. Left on Caselli to No. 101.
23. Right to ascend Clover Lane Stairway and alley up to 19th St.
24. Cross 19th St., and ascend the narrow stairway and steep trail back up to the Kite Hill Open Space and your beginning.

(Continued from page 227)

WALK FACTS

Mind the traffic around the stairs up to Tank Hill as the turn is blind and drivers sometimes speed through here.

There are no trails or paved paths up to Tank Hill, only stairs.

When Mount Olympus is clear of obstructions, it has an unequaled 360-degree view of San Francisco and farther east across the Bay.

Bus Routes & Parking

PUBLIC TRANSPORTATION: MUNI Bus #37 Corbett. For MUNI bus information, call 311 (outside San Francisco, call 415-701-2311).

PARKING: There is metered street parking available; metered parking is usually available for up to an hour, and free street parking is usually allowed for up to two hours. But also look for street-cleaning times posted in the neighborhood to avoid getting ticketed or towed.

WALK 27 DESCRIPTION

◢ The highlights of this walk are detailed in Walks 17–20. Quick-step instructions for Walk 27 run you through the course, hopping you forever forward from hill to hill like a bunny. But as you reach each hilltop, take a moment to enjoy the view, catch your breath, and find out a little bit about what's underfoot.

◢ Kite Hill, formerly named Solari Hill after a farmer who grazed his cattle on the hill, is your first hop, and was once part of "Nobby" Clarke's Water Works property above Clayton. This space provides a well-tended garden for bees, birds, and people alike. This area, of course, also benefits from the kindness of neighbors and their attention to maintaining the trail and planted areas.

◢ Tank Hill, your second hop, is named for the Spring Valley Water Works water tank that adorned it. See two bridges at once, and consider the fact that you are on a panoramic hilltop in the city. Tank Hill Park is a rocky outcropping defining the north side of Twin Peaks, with cliffs that are footed by houses below. Kite Hill is visible from the top of Tank Hill, just to the northwest.

To walk alone in London is the greatest rest.
> —*The Diary of Virginia Woolf*

◢ Mount Olympus, your third hop now enshrined in condominiums and closely packed-in town homes, remains the geographic center of the city. Unfortunately the views from this hilltop are now filled in with urban development. But back in 1887, before he became mayor, and as a gift to the city of San Francisco, Adolph Sutro placed a great monument, a lady liberty, named *The Triumph of Light,* here to watch over us. She was unveiled to an enthusiastic crowd gathered to celebrate the greatness of San Francisco, at the intersection of 16th and Ashbury, which is now filled in with housing. Local dignitaries passed around cigars, and schoolchildren from all across the city attended the event.

◢ Corona Heights (Rock Hill) is our fourth and last hop, made up of leftover crags from the Gray Brothers Brick Factory. From this hill's rocky perch, you can see the closest representation of Daniel Burnham's vision

Mount Olympus   *Mary Burk*

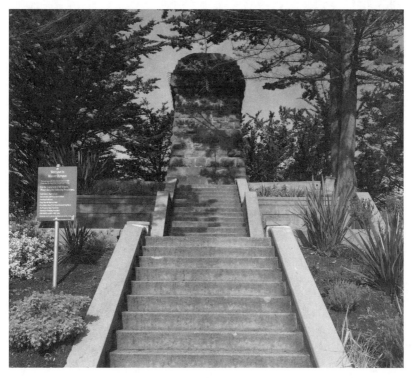

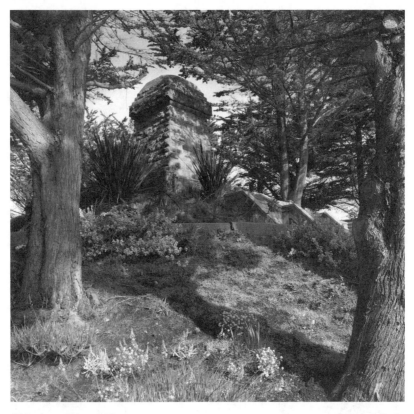

Side view of Mount Olympus   *Mary Burk*

(as he imagined it in his City Beautiful plan) of the view down Market St. to the Ferry Building—wide and expansive.

Further Rambling

If you want additional information about the Corona Heights and Golden Gate Heights neighborhoods, as well as many of the other streets and highlights on the Four Hills route, refer to Walks 17–20 (Walk 20, Eureka Valley, for Kite Hill; Walk 17, Twin Peaks Foothills, for Tank Hill; Walk 18, Upper Market, for Mt. Olympus; and Walk 19, Corona Heights). For those sections not covered in detail elsewhere in the book, enjoy discovering what catches your eye as you experience the walk.

Jazz & Beyond

Sunnyside

Some walks feel bouncy, some feel fettered and bound, and others feel as though they will never end. The best walks have a lilt to them. Adah has always designed her walks so that they have a rhythm, a feeling for the terrain, foliage, rocks, and rooftops.

Musicians throughout the ages have composed music relating to their environment. Beethoven did that beautifully in his *Sixth Symphony*, Vivaldi in the *Four Seasons*, Art Tatum in his *Lullaby of the Leaves*, Herbie Mann in *A Dance at the Rise of the Moon*, and Bobby Hutcherson in *Highway 1*. Even children make up songs about their environment through their everyday activities—jumping rope, shooting marbles, and picking blackberries along a hillside. Adults hum songs describing the physical work they are engaged in. So it seems natural that to think and move to the music of a walk. While neither Adah nor I can compose a jazz piece, she decided that it would be fun to create a walk inspired by jazz.

The Sunnyside neighborhood is wedged between Balboa Park and Glen Canyon Park. The homes are small but well taken care of, and all of the front yards are stunning with succulents of varied colors and concentric designs. No. 12 Baden is an earthquake shack from 1907. No. 163 Mangels and No. 330 Congo date to 1899. No. 257 Joost was built in 1900. This jazz route has a contrast that translates into lovely musical harmonies.

WALK FACTS

Served by the Balboa Park and Glen Park MUNI and BART stations, this neighborhood is also very close to San Francisco City College.

Dorothy Erskine Park is also nearby; see directions for rambling further at the end of the walk.

When land developer Behrend Joost advertised lots for sale in this neighborhood, the slogan read, "The largest and most important subdivision ever placed on the San Francisco market."

The Sunnyside Conservatory puts on events and classes, as does the Sunnyside Neighborhood Association. The latter also organizes street and park cleanup meetings for volunteers.

Renovated in 2007, the Sunnyside Playground features a much improved park. Look for colorful play equipment, a sandbox, water fountain, merry-go-round, tennis and basketball courts, a large grassy area, and picnic tables.

Bus Routes & Parking

PUBLIC TRANSPORTATION: MUNI Bus #23 Monterey and #36 Teresita. For MUNI bus information, call 311 (outside San Francisco, call 415-701-2311).

PARKING: There is metered street parking available; metered parking is usually available for up to an hour, and free street parking is usually allowed for up to two hours. But also look for street-cleaning times posted in the neighborhood to avoid getting ticketed or towed.

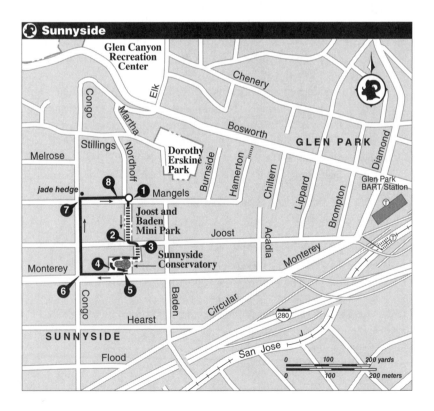

QUICK-STEP INSTRUCTIONS

1. Begin at Mangels across from Nordhoff. Descend stairway into Joost and Baden Mini Park to Joost.

2. Cross Joost. Continue left for a few yards.

3. Enter arched gate to Sunnyside Conservatory Park, between Nos. 233 and 241 Joost. Descend groups of stairways to the conservatory.

4. Walk around conservatory building. Descend stairway to Monterey Blvd.

5. Right to Congo.

6. Right and continue up the hill to Mangels.

7. Cross street at Mangels to the jade hedge.

8. Continue to Baden and your beginning.

WALK 28 DESCRIPTION

Begin at Mangels and Nordhoff, next to a vacant lot. When a group of us were exploring the neighborhood in 2006, the house on this lot was leaning heavily into the house next to it. Groups of neighbors, trucks, and workers were gathered around it. Three hours later when we walked back to check on it, there was no longer a house there. The new owner had bought it at a court auction with the warnings "as is" and "enter at your own risk," and when he was working on the foundation, it gave way, crashing into the house next to it. The poignancy of the pain and distress of the event permeates this walk. Adah always compares it to hearing the saxophone and trumpet wails in Terence Blanchard's *A Tale of God's Will (A Requiem for Katrina)*.

Next to the lot, on the right, a sign reads, "Joost & Baden Mini Park Stairway." The stairway leads us on a short descent into a garden of succulents, asters, geraniums, sages of different colors, and shrubs and trees—a fairyland park. It is a surprise. Curving corners and greenery edging the curbstones give an additional sense of privacy and comfort. Continue walking through the levels of the garden to Joost. This seems to be the perfect place for the sparkling piano of Art Tatum playing *Humoresque*.

At the mini park sign, turn left and walk a few yards to the iron gate between Nos. 233 and 241 Joost. Descend the stairway into the Sunnyside Conservatory Park. A two-story octagonal structure dating from the 1890s, the conservatory was built on a subdivided dairy farm lot. When the Van Beck family bought the property in 1919, the conservatory was covered with foliage; they discovered it only by looking for their lost dog who was trapped inside!

◢ Interest in the conservatory was ignited in 1973 when new owners applied for a permit to demolish the building. The Sunnyside Neighborhood Association was organized, and the building was given Landmark Status No. 78. Finally after many mishaps (you can read about the history posted on the building wall to the right), the Friends of Sunnyside Conservatory was formed in 1999. They sponsor workdays, art classes, and community events. The city was impressed by the excellent plans the association pulled together, as was the Department of Recreation and Parks, and the many volunteers' gigantic efforts were eventually rewarded with $4 million in 2006 for renovation work. On December 5, 2009, the grand reopening of the Sunnyside Conservatory took place. The two-story, high-ceilinged center octagon basks in natural light from the windows surrounding it. This large interior room, ordinarily locked, is available for rental and special functions.

◢ Continue around the structure where a variety of succulents and ferns, mallows, geraniums, African lilies, and impatiens have been planted. Here too is a magnolia tree and some heritage palms, Canary Island, Chilean wine, and Norfolk Island, all of which enrich the experience of the conservatory park tour and its flowering beauty.

◢ A special feature of the park is the Menagerie Project designed by Scott Constable and Ene Osteraas-Constable of Wowhaus, a well-known and celebrated art and sculpture team. A doorknob in the shape of a squirrel and other fanciful creatures are at ease around the grounds among the plants and embedded in the concrete. The Friends of Sunnyside Conservatory feels that the park's revival far exceeds their expectations. When it was at its lowest point of disrepair, it was hard to imagine that it would one day reach its present state of splendor. The conservatory is the perfect building and setting for the Haydn *Piano Sonata in F Major* played by Vladimir Horowitz.

◢ Descend the stairway to Monterey Blvd. Turn right on Monterey, and continue to Congo. There is a fine view of San Bruno Mountain and the radio towers at the corner and as you walk up the right side of Congo to Joost. Continue to Mangels, and cross the street to the jade hedge on the corner. The hedge, full of blooms, is a perfect example of having the right plants, in right weather, in just the right growing

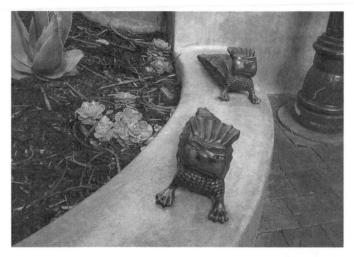

Menagerie Project   *Tony Holiday*

conditions. At the corner ahead, breaking through the wood fence, is a deformed tree. As you walk toward Baden, a multicolored stone wall and terraced garden come into view. Continue toward them to your beginning.

Further Rambling

To enjoy Dorothy Erskine Park, head one block north on Nordhoff, and then turn right on Stillings; the park is about two blocks east. The park land was acquired by the city in 1997, and named after the Bay Area environmentalist, Dorothy Erskine, founder of the Greenbelt Alliance, and a founding member of SPUR (San Francisco Planning and Urban Research Association, a nonprofit urban planning and good government organization). Erskine worked to find housing for the poor, promote urban and regional planning for parks and open-space areas, and also preserve farmland areas in San Francisco, San Jose, and Oakland.

Past, Present & Future

The Blue Greenway

Although this book focuses on neighborhood walks in the hilly sections of San Francisco, the newly developing Mission Bay neighborhood in the southeastern area of the city includes residences and businesses of interest; the University of California, Mission Creek campus; and the Blue Greenway. A community has begun to coalesce.

The Blue Greenway is a 13-mile waterfront trail along the San Francisco Bay shoreline that comprises the city's portion of the Bay Trail. The trail connects existing green spaces to new ones and links land and water resources so that people can enjoy nature and recreational activities. It is exciting to watch the Blue Greenway progressing toward fulfillment of these goals.

Corinne Woods, a resident of the Mission Creek neighborhood, has lived in her floating home since 1987 and is an activist for Mission Bay and the Port of San Francisco's waterfront planning. When the Mission Bay Park system is complete, approximately 49 acres of open space will be available for use by the general public.

In 1996, Isabel Wade organized the Neighborhood Parks Alliance, the city's foremost park advocacy group. In 2005, the group launched the Blue Greenway Initiative, and the mayor created a task force. Woods teamed up with Wade and has since been working as chief advocate for the Blue Greenway. When Woods walked us through her route, it was obvious that she had refined it during many years of exploring.

WALK FACTS

Walking the Embarcadero in different weather presents different challenges. Bring sunglasses if it's sunny, since the expanses of road and sidewalk next to the sparkling waterfront can blind you. As night falls, the temperature can drop quickly along the Bay, and the wind can pick up too, so dress and plan accordingly.

The Embarcadero Promenade is a favorite of joggers and walkers. The shops inside the Ferry Building and the farmers' market (held Tuesdays, Thursdays, and Saturdays) offer plenty of gourmet choices. Look for foodies and marathoners alike.

The Exploratorium at Piers 15 and 17 is a museum of science, art, and human perception (open Tuesday–Sunday, 10 a.m.–5 p.m.). Children and adults can touch, look at, and listen to the exhibits. High school students in the explainer program are available to answer questions. The museum was founded by the late physicist Dr. Frank Oppenheimer and his wife, Jackie.

Bus Routes & Parking

PUBLIC TRANSPORTATION: MUNI Metro T Line, F Embarcadero, N Judah, and Bus #1 California. If you end at King St., your options include: Bus #10 Townsend at the corner of Townsend and 3rd St.; Bus #30 Stockton, #45 Union, #47 Van Ness, and T Line, all at Townsend and 4th St. near the Caltrain Station; and Muni Bus N Line (weekdays only) at King and 4th St. For MUNI bus or metro information, call 311 (outside San Francisco, call 415-701-2311).

PARKING: Parking in this area is minimal and expensive. Take public transportation instead.

WALK 29 DESCRIPTION

◢ We begin our walk at Rincon Park on the Embarcadero between Howard and Folsom. *Cupid's Span,* an audacious, unconventional sculpture by Claes Oldenburg and Coosje van Bruggen, is placed in the center of the park for all to see and react to—what a greeting! You may feel like dancing around it. The park was developed by Gap, Inc., and the sculpture was commissioned by Donald and Doris Fisher, the company's founders.

◢ Walk along the Embarcadero past Red's Java House at Pier 30. It opened in 1923 as a lunchroom for longshoremen and waterfront workers. As you continue to Townsend and 2nd, you will see elegant interpretive signposts listing pertinent historic information about San Francisco's early waterfront years. Bloody Thursday occurred in the area between Market and 2nd on July 5, 1934, during the International Longshoremen's Workers Union strike, one of the bloodiest union strikes in US history.

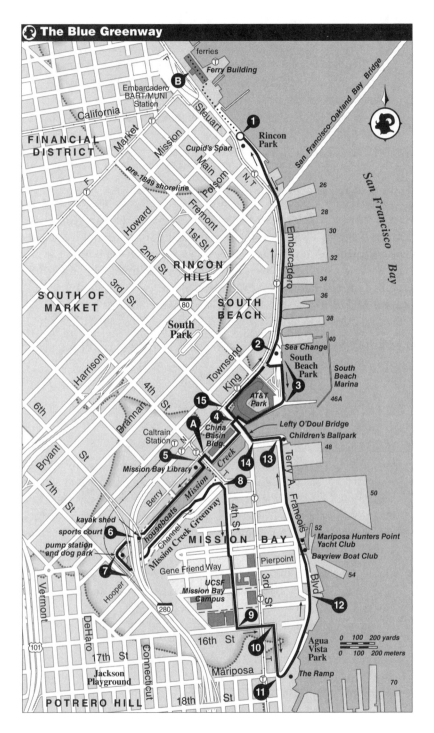

The Blue Greenway

QUICK-STEP INSTRUCTIONS

1. Begin at Rincon Park on the Embarcadero between Howard and Folsom at the *Cupid's Span* sculpture. Walk along the Embarcadero to Pier 40.

2. Continue to 2nd and Townsend to the *Sea Change* sculpture. Walk around South Beach Park, South Beach Harbor, and South Beach Yacht Club.

3. Walk around South Beach Marina and behind AT&T Park to 3rd at Lefty O'Doul Bridge.

4. Cross 3rd at crosswalk. Continue on promenade along Mission Creek to 4th.

5. Cross 4th at crosswalk. Continue on Mission Creek past the floating homes.

6. Walk to the path by the kayak storage building. Continue around the sports fields.

7. Bear left on path around dog park and sewer pump station building. Turn left on path along other side of Mission Creek.

8. At 4th St. turn right. Continue along UCSF buildings and to 16th.

9. Turn left and cross 3rd to Illinois.

10. Right on Illinois to Mariposa.

11. Left on Mariposa to Terry Francois Blvd., and turn left.

12. Continue on Terry Francois past Pier 48.

13. Bear left at China Basin. Continue to 3rd at the bridge.

14. Right on 3rd.

15. Right on King. If you wish to end your walk here, see the public transit information for this walk. Otherwise, continue to the Embarcadero and your beginning.

Walking is the best possible exercise. You should not permit yourself even to think while you walk, but divert yourself by the objects surrounding you.

—Thomas Jefferson, in a letter to a friend, 1790

◢ At South Beach Park, Mark di Suvero's sculpture *Sea Change* stands taller than anything else around. The 700-berth, fully occupied marina has been in operation since 1986.

◢ We continue around the marina, past the South Beach Yacht Club, to AT&T Park, home to the San Francisco Giants, which opened in April 2000 and has undergone several name changes. There are sidewalk

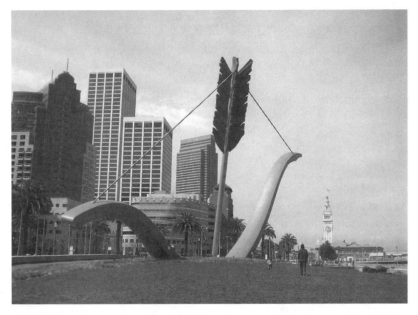

Cupid's Span   *Tony Holiday*

insets of Giants events in the walkway, featuring retired Giants players along King, along with the Wall of Fame. Closer to the Lefty
O'Doul Bridge is the free viewing area—standing room only—where
people can watch the game in "The Cove," named for Willie McCovey.
Through spaces in the fence under an archway, the viewing area is
democratically run. Each person is allowed to watch three innings and
then gives up their space to someone else.

◢ Continue from AT&T Park to 3rd and the Lefty O'Doul Bridge, and
cross at the crosswalk. Now we are in the China Basin area, named
for the China clippers of the Pacific Mail Steamship Company line,
which docked here at Steamboat Point during the 1860s. Walk on the
promenade along Mission Creek in front of the dominating China
Basin Building. At 4th, cross at the crosswalk.

◢ Cities continually move. San Francisco is stretching out toward the
southeast, building up parkways and a clean Mission Creek. Along
the main streets of King, Townsend, and 4th, grocery stores have
appeared, as well as bakeries, a special coffeehouse that prepares individual servings of fresh coffee, and other specialty and sidewalk-front
stores. New housing developed around the ballpark includes condos

and low-cost to middle-class rentals. The Mission Bay Branch Library occupies the first floor of the 400-unit senior living center at the corner of King and 4th. As you continue, the Mission Creek Marina comes into view. The floating homes are painted in various colors that contribute a feeling of neighborliness. They are a community of activists, they love living near the water, and they keep it clean; the grounds around their houses have plantings, and many of them also work their plots in the community garden.

◢ At the kayak storage building, continue around the sports fields by the volleyball court. Walk left on the path around the dog park and sewer pump station building. At the end of the path, turn left to walk back along the other side of Mission Creek.

◢ A community garden is on the right. Walk along Channel St. toward the Mission Creek Greenway. This area is slated to be parkland, additional condos, and apartment buildings. Continue through the park to 4th.

◢ At 4th turn right, and continue along an area that was once occupied by warehouses and a railroad yard and is now the University of California, San Francisco (UCSF) Mission Bay campus. UCSF began

Embarcadero interpretive panel   *Tony Holiday*

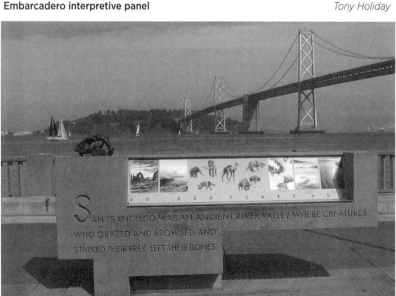

opening laboratories and classrooms at this location in 2003, and several other facilities have opened since that time. The children's and women's specialties and cancer hospital complex are being constructed in 2014 and will open in early 2015.

◢ Continue to 16th, turn left and cross 3rd. Walk to Illinois, and turn right continuing to Mariposa. At Mariposa, turn left, and continue to Terry Francois Blvd. After turning left on Terry Francois, continue past the Ramp Restaurant, a very happy place. Everyone enjoys lunching along the water. Then we pass Agua Vista Park, and Pier 52 with its historic railroad ferry ramp, the Bayview Boat Club, the new public boat launch ramp, the Mariposa Hunters Point Yacht Club, and Pier 50, and Pier 48.

◢ At the end, to the right are a children's ballpark and a Willie McCovey sculpture. Continue left at China Basin Cove, walking along the baseball sculptures, to 3rd, and turn right onto King to the front entrance of the AT&T Park. The Willie Mays sculpture is on the right.

◢ If you wish to end your walk here, check the public transit details listed for this walk. If not, continue on King St. to the Embarcadero, and turn left to your beginning. (And, yes, level walking is different from stairway walking.)

The Good View

Upper Haight

There's nothing more rejuvenating than a San Francisco stairway walk. When you throw in some twists, a few turns, and a surprising, stupendous view, who could ask for anything more? On this walk through the Upper Haight, you will enjoy a small taste of the terraces, a pleasant amble through the best parts of Buena Vista Park, and a large gulp of a view to reward you for your efforts.

In 2011, the City of San Francisco dedicated a stairway to Adah Bakalinsky, the queen of San Francisco stairways. The city pays tribute to stairways on an ongoing basis by partnering with neighborhood groups like 16th Avenue and Hidden Garden Steps to improve the beauty of the staircases themselves. And because of Adah and her love of stairways, Gavin Newsom (mayor of San Francisco at the time and now lieutenant governor of California) declared March 2, 2006, Stairway Day in her honor. The great walks that Adah has shared over the last three decades (through now eight editions of this book) are a secret pleasure in San Francisco that only savvy tourists and excellent locals seem to share.

But this walk skirts many other notable areas, each connected or nearby peeking in and between the hilly neighborhoods that surround the hill Adolph Sutro dubbed the center of the city. This walk starts with the lady of the stairs, takes you up over hill and dale, turns you around a mansion hairpin, then spins you back for a little bit more of the park's good views and hills and the houses surrounding it. Let's begin.

WALK FACTS

The Upper Haight shopping district from Masonic to Stanyan still features many 1960s counterculture and hippie outlets for clothing, paraphernalia, and souvenirs. It also offers neighborhood shops like Whole Foods, Mendel's Art and Fabrics, Robert's Hardware, and Amoeba Records.

(Continued on page 248)

QUICK-STEP INSTRUCTIONS

1. Begin at No. 1 Broderick near Waller. Take the Adah Bakalinsky Stairway on the left up to Buena Vista Terrace East.

2. Left on Buena Vista Terrace East. Walk uphill to Duboce, and use the crosswalk into Buena Vista Park. Enter the park by taking the grand staircase; stay left.

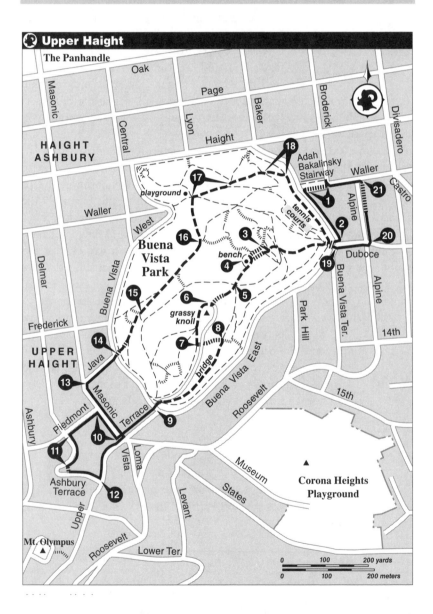

3. Take the paved path straight ahead into the park. When it splits, continue up the wooden stairs, continuing up either left or right.

4. Take the wooden stairs up the hill behind the wooden bench. Follow the dirt path on the left (east) side of the hill. When the dirt path becomes paved again, continue forward.

5. From the WPA fountain, it's 41 more steps to the top.

6. Walk past the grass circle to its other end, and proceed toward a map of the park. Before you reach the map, turn left. Follow the nearby path down to a wooden stairway at the back side of Buena Vista Park.

7. From the top of the wooden stairway, walk down to the newer stairs. Proceed down one flight to the wooden footbridge.

8. Take the footbridge, and hold onto the handrails. Once the path becomes paved again, continue down the hill and out of the park.

9. Cross the street onto Upper Terrace at the intersection of Buena Vista East and Buena Vista West.

10. Cross onto Masonic, and walk down one block to Piedmont. Left on Piedmont, and walk one more block east.

11. Left on Ashbury Terrace, following the curve up the street toward the hairpin turn. At the top of the circular staircase, go left back up to Upper Terrace.

12. Take Upper Terrace back to Masonic. Walk down Masonic, past Piedmont one more block to Java St., turn right.

13. Walk one block on Java to Buena Vista West.

14. Cross Buena Vista West back into the park, take the tiny wood steps, and stay left to enter the forest side of Buena Vista.

15. Soon you enter a wooded grove; keep heading east on the dirt path that soon becomes paved.

16. Stay left as you circumnavigate the north side of the park. Walk the lower path heading north and toward the children's playground.

17. When the paved path takes another turn up, stay right, but don't turn upward back into the park. Take the paved path down to the park's inner, lower promenade with diamond brick designs.

18. Walk up the promenade, and head up Buena Vista East, passing the Adah Bakalinsky Stairway. Stay on the path in the park to Duboce.

19. Cross out of the park to walk down Duboce heading east.

20. Take Duboce one block to Alpine, turn left, and walk down on the east side of the street.

21. Walk one block down Alpine to Waller. Turn left on Waller, and walk one block west to your beginning.

(Continued from page 245)

The Haight Street Fair, or Haight-Ashbury Fair, is held in June, and 2014 marks its 37th year. Music stages are set up at both Masonic and Stanyan, and more than 200 vendors sell food, crafts, and other services during the event.

Although it technically begins narrowly in the Panhandle, Golden Gate Park really starts at the end of Haight St. at Stanyan. Near this park entrance, you can walk by a small pond and then under a stalagmite-designed underpass to Sharon Meadow (Hippie Hill) and the Carousel.

Bus Routes & Parking

PUBLIC TRANSPORTATION: MUNI Bus #71 Haight, #43 Masonic, #33 Stanyan (in walking distance), and #24 Divisadero (in walking distance). For MUNI bus information, call 311 (outside San Francisco, call 415-701-2311).

PARKING: There is metered street parking available; metered parking is usually available for up to an hour, and free street parking is usually allowed for up to two hours. But also look for street-cleaning times posted in the neighborhood to avoid getting ticketed or towed.

WALK 30 DESCRIPTION

◢ Begin at No. 1 Broderick near Waller. Up the hill to Buena Vista Terrace East, there is a ramp on the right, and the Adah Bakalinsky Stairway on the left. In between there is a wild, terraced garden. Count the steps up—you can make it to 90. Turn left on Buena Vista Terrace East.

◢ Walk uphill to Duboce, and use the crosswalk into Buena Vista Park. Enter the park by taking the grand staircase near the green sign; stay to the left. Take the paved path straight ahead up into the park. (The path to the right takes you to the tennis courts.)

◢ When the path splits, continue up the wood stairs straight ahead. Near the top of the wood stairs past the first landing, stay left and approach a green bench ahead of you, facing east.

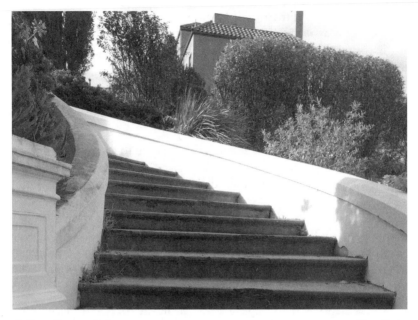

Ashbury Terrace Stairway   *Mary Burk*

◢ Now take a seat on the bench dedicated to Tina Smith Coyne of San Francisco (1957–2001):

> *Rest here—weary walker*
> *Enjoy the view with me.*
> *I found peace—so shall ye.*

◢ After enjoying the view to the east, take the wooden stairs up to the top of the hill behind you. Follow the path on the left or east side of the hill.

◢ You will see a knee-high sprinkler atop a stone brick pyramid. What looks like a sprinkler monument is actually a nonworking drinking fountain installed by the Works Progress Administration (WPA). Hopefully, it too can someday be restored. Continue up the paved path straight ahead.

◢ Near the apex of the park, the paved path once again has stairs, fashioned out of the same stones that line the path's low rock walls below you and the drainage trench to your right. You climb 41 more steps to get to the top, which has another beautiful view.

◢ When you reach the top of Buena Vista Park, you'll notice that the view isn't as nice as Tina's, but it's still welcoming. The grassy knoll is encircled by stones, and this respite above the Haight St. tourists is framed by pine and cypress trees.

◢ From the top, walk past the grass circle to its other end, and proceed down another paved path toward a map of the park. Just before you reach the map, turn left. Follow the shaded path downward.

◢ Now take a small wooden stairway downward to cross a larger paved path, toward a stone entrance near a green "No Littering" sign. From the top of this stairway, walk down the newer stairs lined by metal handrails, and you will see the new reinforced stairs whose risers are covered with traction grips. Proceed one flight down to the wooden footbridge. On the footbridge, hold onto the wooden handrails on your right. Stop for a view of Corona Heights (Rock Hill) and the Randall Museum below you. Once the footbridge becomes a paved path again, continue down the hill and out of the park.

◢ Cross the street onto Upper Terrace, at the intersection of Buena Vista East and Buena Vista West. Note the brick house at the corner of Upper Terrace and Masonic. The sign over its driveway reads "Le Petit Chateau des Cavaliers"—"the small house of jumpers." Still, you are surrounded by many mansions happily cozied up next to one another upon the hill.

◢ Cross onto Masonic, and walk down one block to Piedmont. Turn left on Piedmont, and walk one more block east. The houses and street wind together here tightly. Your next turn reveals the hairpin turn.

◢ Now turn left on Ashbury Terrace, and follow the curve up the street to a shortcut around the hairpin turn. In the middle of the Ashbury Terrace hairpin is a grand buttery yellow staircase. At the top of the circular staircase, turn left, and head back up to Upper Terrace. A pirouette and we go in a new direction, in search of—coffee?

◢ Go left again to walk down Masonic, walk past Piedmont one block, and turn right onto Java St. In 1892, the San Francisco Fire Department's Anza Vista location was served by Chemical Engine Wagon No. 7, whose quarters were at Java and Masonic. The houses now bear little resemblance to that day, though most were built on this street in the decade after the firehouse was moved.

◢ At the end of Java, you again face Buena Vista Park, and you are on Buena Vista West. Cross Buena Vista West, and take the tiny wood stairway steps back into the park. Stay on the path to the left. The path to the left takes you through another shaded glen and then turns into a dirt path. Remember to stay left. In the glen below, you will see a dog run and a sign guiding you down to the area. Keep walking past it for now on the paved path. Stay on the upper path, and begin heading north.

◢ As you enjoy the shady redwoods all around, you then come to a children's playground. Continue past the playground, and stay right on the level path, which now begins to take you east. However, when the paved path forks, stay right; don't take the path that climbs back up into the park. Instead take the narrow, paved path down to the park's inner stroll, a sidewalk decorated with diamond brick inlaid designs running down the middle of the concrete promenade around Buena Vista East.

◢ As you stroll along the diamond promenade past Adah's stairway and up toward Duboce, you'll see great views to the east where you entered the park at the grand staircase. Here you walk past homes that were once the palaces of sugar barons, silent film stars, and US ambassadors. Consider Rudolph Valentino out for a morning stroll, elegance personified, making sure to watch his step down the same steep block of Duboce you too now descend.

◢ Walk down Duboce one block to Alpine, and turn left, first crossing to the right or east side of Alpine. Here you find a favorite stairway necessity. When the steepness of a hill requires cutting steps into the sidewalk itself, walkers at least have surer footing options. Walk down Alpine's sidewalk stairway one block to Waller.

◢ Turn left on Waller, and walk one block west to return to your beginning.

Further Rambling

You can connect this walk to Walks 17 (Twin Peaks), 18 (Upper Market), and 19 (Corona Heights). Connect to Walk 19 by doubling back to Buena Vista Terrace at this walk's endpoint, and then walk east toward Roosevelt. Since Walk 27 is four hills on its own, it's a connection for only the heartiest of walkers.

Nearby neighborhoods include Cole Valley, Castro St., and the Upper and Lower Haight. Each has its own unique and friendly ways. Haight is divided in half at Divisadero; trundle on.

The Serendipity Slipknot

Dogpatch

Like a slipknot, this walk can easily be untied
or wound back together again, depending on how
your day unfolds. Its serendipitous nature led Adah
and I along; each step felt brand new because we didn't
know exactly what we would find. But as we gained our
bearings, the neighborhood began to take shape around us,
and we discovered interesting sites, happy accidental signposts—
which are just a few of the accidental highlights we enjoyed while
ambling and getting turned about. Explore the Dogpatch neighborhood after this walk and see where serendipity takes you.

Dogpatch lies in the southeastern portion of San Francisco, skirting
the eastern edge of Potrero Hill. Our own bona fide flatlands, Dogpatch
includes the city's largest collection of 19th- and early-20th-century workers' cottages, and the City of San Francisco recognized the neighborhood
as a historic district for these homes and buildings in 2003.

The neighborhood has a colorful history and holds a unique place
in the growth of industrial economics for San Francisco. Dogpatch is
the original slang name for the area, here at Potrero Point, which used
to sit alongside its neighboring community on Irish Hill, gone now since
World War I. (The name is not a nod to Al Capp's *Li'l Abner* comic strip,
which refers to Dogpatch, Kentucky.) Much of the land in Dogpatch near
the waterfront was taken up by the Union Iron Works shipyard, which
still stands at 1060 Tennessee St. The neighborhood, however, was truly
defined by the work performed here, and the laborers who lived near the
business that employed them. By the late 1860s, this area had already
developed into the city's densest industrial center and employed thousands of skilled craftsmen.

The neighborhood was first established by Irish, Scottish, and Eng-
lish immigrants. Later waves of immigrants settling in Dogpatch included
Italians, Scandinavians, Mexicans, Dust Bowl migrants, and African
Americans.

The neighborhood was spared from the fire damage that swept
away Victorian homes south of Market after the 1906 earthquake, mainly

because it was so isolated, and connected to downtown only by a wooden bridge running along the side of the Bay (on what is now 3rd St.). Mission Bay and the Islais Inlet separated Dogpatch from much of the disaster. In many ways, the urban community in Dogpatch resembles what it was a century ago, in part because of the efforts of the Dogpatch Neighborhood Association formed in 1998, which engage with city agencies to support urban planning and historic preservation. What was once an industrial suburb on the other side of the marshlands has become a modern vibrant community that is reinventing itself while preserving its past and welcoming new neighbors as the area continues to grow and improve.

WALK FACTS

This walk is relatively flat, but on a sunny day, you can get a sunburn faster in this neighborhood than in others due to its proximity to the Bay. Wear sunscreen if it's sunny.

Progress Park, under Interstate 280 at 23rd and Indiana, is a new community volunteer park. Work on it is managed through donations by the Dogpatch Neighborhood Association; it has been recognized by the *San Francisco Chronicle* and won a San Francisco Community Challenge Grant. Visit it and see what's sprouting.

Dogpatch artists hold open studios on weekends in April and October. Contact **dogpatchart.com/tag/open-studios** for more information on specific weekend dates in 2014 and beyond.

Bus Routes & Parking

PUBLIC TRANSPORTATION: MUNI KT–Ingleside and 3rd (light rail, outbound for Balboa Park). For MUNI bus or Metro information, call 311 (outside San Francisco, call 415-701-2311).

PARKING: Most of the street parking is metered; metered parking is usually for up to an hour, and free street parking is usually allowed for up to two hours. Look for street-cleaning times posted in the neighborhood to avoid getting ticketed or towed.

WALK 31 DESCRIPTION

◢ Begin near the T line exit, at Mariposa and 3rd St. Cross 3rd, and walk east (toward the Bay). Walk one more block down Mariposa to Illinois, where a few peek-a-boo looks at the Bay come into view. Turn right, and walk down Illinois two blocks south to 20th St. and the Dogpatch Café, which houses a gallery.

◢ When Adah and I first scouted this walk, the café was hosting a pop-up gallery for the Museum of Craft and Design. The museum opened in April 2013 at its permanent address (No. 2569 3rd) and is worth a visit. For now, continue toward the Bay, just beyond some large fences and the dark baked-red brick buildings to your left.

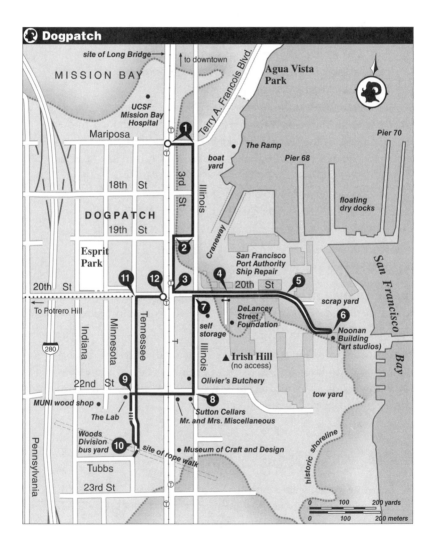

QUICK-STEP INSTRUCTIONS

1. Start at Embarcadero Station (or any underground station going inbound on the KT line). Disembark at 3rd and Mariposa. Cross 3rd, and walk one more block east to Illinois. Then turn right, and walk three blocks south to Illinois and 20th.

2. Right on 19th, and left on 3rd to 20th and Illinois.

3. Left on 20th, and walk east toward the San Francisco Port Authority Ship Repair (20th and Illinois).

4. Right toward signs for DeLancey. Leave the outreach center, and continue east on 20th.

5. Continue east toward Pier 70, the Noonan Building, and the artists' studios.

6. Turn around, and go west on 20th back to Illinois. Walk south down Illinois around Dogpatch Self Storage and Irish Hill. Continue south to Sutton Cellars at 601 22nd. Head west on 22nd. Continue south on Illinois for one block, toward Olivier's Butchery at No. 1074.

7. Return back over 3rd to continue west on 20th.

8. Turn left on Tennessee to arrive at the Chocolate Lab.

9. Continue south down Tennessee on the right. Use the stairs between the cottages at No. 1108.

10. Where Tennessee ends at a ramped sidewalk, take the sidewalk switchover to its intersection with Tubbs. Loop back to Tennessee to head north. Walk about three blocks to 20th.

11. Walk past the overpass from Dogpatch to Potrero Hill (pay close attention to traffic if you extend your walk to the west).

12. Continue right on 20th back to 3rd. The inbound KT line stops at 3rd and 20th, or you can walk back to 18th and 3rd to your beginning.

◢ Walk another block east on 20th past Illinois. Continue west toward the San Francisco Port Authority Ship Repair, just past Illinois. The day we visited was a bright, sunny day in September, yet we could not see the water for the ships covered in rust and towering above us at street level, with 12-foot barbwire fences separating us from the water. It is very hard to tell you are standing only 2 feet above sea level and that the Bay is just about 20 yards away. The buildings lining this block of 20th are the former Steel Works company. Since it closed, their elegant entrance stairs made of marble and flanked by white cornices serve as skateboard ramps and a place for occasional passersby to stop and rest.

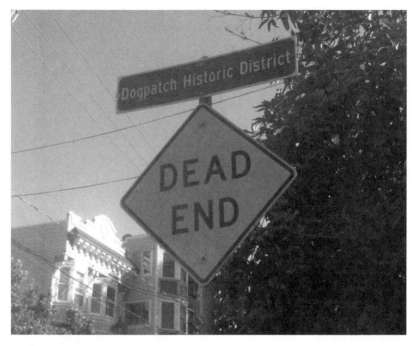

Dead end in Dogpatch   *Mary Burk*

◢ Continue on 20th past abandoned machine works buildings and giant, empty workshops built with red brick and blue-green iron, crumbling quietly under the sun. These are the Steel Works buildings, and you soon reach a gate for "Port Authority Ship Repair" on your left. However, you cannot venture past it without clearance. Going beyond the fence to dip a toe in the Bay would be trespassing, so take a right, and head south down curving 20th. Soon you walk past the DeLancey Street Foundation's Outreach area. The foundation, founded in 1971 in San Francisco, helps former convicts, drug and alcohol users, and other individuals reestablish themselves in their communities through work programs, community housing, and counseling. But the lot adjacent to DeLancey is also private property, and the outreach center is closed to the general public.

◢ Double back from DeLancey to continue walking east on 20th. The wooden building near the end of the street is an artist's studio, where artists rent space and hold open studio shows for the public. The artist Adah and I greeted also echoed the sentiment we felt in the neighborhood—that it's growing and changing. He mentioned that he has seen more and more people in the area every weekend. Soon you reach the Noonan Building at Pier 70, which is one of the last standing wood buildings in the area (and in surprisingly good shape), providing low-rent studios for local artists.

◢ Turn around and return on 20th St. back to Illinois. Development plans for the waterfront have so far spared the best thing you can see from the corner of 20th and Illinois—a tiny green hill. Before Bethlehem Steel moved in, before the Long Bridge was built, and even before the railroads reached this neighborhood, and when ships were the only thing being built in Dogpatch, Irish Hill was a rowdy neighborhood all its own and a very different place. Once a community site of more than 60 cottages, it was a thriving neighborhood made up mostly of single Irish immigrant men.

◢ Irish Hill was taken apart in stages. Prior to World War I, Bethlehem Steel quarried and dynamited most of it to make way for shipyard expansion. And before that, in the late 1800s, Irish Hill was also quarried to help fill in the Bay underneath Long Bridge, which 3rd mainly follows today. Potrero Point's serpentine crest once rose high above the buildings surrounding you and ran across the freeway and all the

Irish Hill   *Mary Burk*

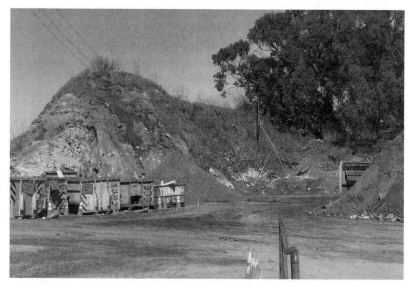

way to Potrero Hill 15 blocks to the west. With the construction of Long Bridge, development quarries removed 100,000 cubic yards of rock and demolished the hill. The cottages were cleared to make way for the railroads, which then also used the rock to fill in a large portion of Mission Bay. All of this earthmoving drastically changed the Bay here and this area's landscape to accommodate railroads, thoroughfares for cars, and deeper ports for ships.

⬛ At the corner of 20th and Illinois is Dogpatch Self Storage, you can see what is left of the serpentine ridge named Irish Hill. It sits behind a chain-link fence and looks like it will soon be razed for who knows what development plan, but I hope this little hill is saved. Continue south on Illinois past the remnants of Irish Hill.

⬛ The neighborhood grows up around you again as you walk away from Irish Hill. At No. 1074 Illinois, Olivier's Butchery offers gourmet cuts of different meats for special order or from the cases on display. The neighborhood shops often organize open-house events and put on barbecues with wine pairings and dessert; many people attend the gatherings, visiting with friends.

⬛ Turn right on 22nd, and notice Sutton Cellars at No. 601. On open house days or during some tasting hours, Sutton Cellars works with Olivier's to supply hamburgers and sausages for community events. Many local businesses participate in the neighborhood open house events; check the Dogpatch Neighborhood Association calendar for more information. Some businesses like Sutton Cellars were previously only open on weekends, but they found that these weekend events have brought them more and more new customers. The area seems to be drawing interest, and Sutton's owners mentioned they were very happy to be part of that evolution.

⬛ We then headed off to visit a nearby chocolate factory, but on the way there, you can decide if you would prefer ice cream. Continue west across 3rd St., and pass the ice-cream shop, Mr. and Mrs. Miscellaneous, at No. 699 22nd. Cross 3rd at Illinois to go west on 22nd. It is clear once you arrive at the Chocolate Lab, a shop created by Recchiuti Confectioners, at No. 601 22nd (at the corner of Tennessee) that you've walked through the real heart of this neighborhood. You have passed a bustling café and several walkers, and now you stand among many original Victorian cottages. This is the Dogpatch historic neighborhood. However, you can still spy a few newer developments farther down Tennessee from this intersection.

◢ Turn left on Tennessee, and head south, walking on the west side of Tennessee. Look for a shaded, four-step stairway in the sidewalk, separating one small cottage from another at No. 1110. Continue south. At No. 1060 Tennessee is the Omega Boys Club, who created the Alive and Free program, which provides educational outreach to troubled young people. This building was also the first children's schoolhouse in Dogpatch, named the Irving M. Scott School, built in 1895. In the 1880s, Irving M. Scott served as the head of the Union Iron Works shipyard located at Pier 70.

◢ Tennessee ends at a ramped sidewalk. Tennessee and Tubbs only intersect because Tennessee continues south after it hitches over about 30 feet to the west at Tubbs. The Tubbs Cordage Company operated in this area from the 1850s until 1962. Brothers Alfred and Hiram Tubbs hailed from New Hampshire but soon bought land here in the Potrero area and across the Bay in Oakland. They built hotels in San Francisco south of Market Street, but their main business was supplying rope to ships up and down the West Coast and internationally.

◢ The Tubbs brothers also helped found the Mountain View Cemetery in Oakland, where their family vault is located. But in San Francisco, all that remains of the Tubbs Cordage Company is a street name. The Tubbs company buildings were demolished, and the land now serves as a bus yard for MUNI.

◢ Turn around at Tubbs, and head north on Tennessee to 20th. Look left to see an on-ramp clambering slowly up toward Potrero Hill, just over Interstate 280 to the west; this is 20th. Try to imagine a mossy green range of serpentine hills rising gradually up the on-ramp, the lost hills from Irish behind you to Potrero Hill beyond, and you will realize just how much the landscape has changed. On the way back down Tennessee heading north, you pass a number of print and ink shops, part of Dogpatch's creative core that developers thankfully want to preserve.

◢ Turn right on 20th, and walk back to 3rd (another stop on the MUNI KT line) and 20th. Although this walk has you meander down one path and then backtrack to try another, it's good practice to take a peek around here and there. Continuing north on Illinois, we saw two more professional print studios on this quiet neighborhood street.

◢ To your left as you walk north on Illinois, look over the overpass. It's only a 15-minute walk to Potrero Hill heading west, but for now, continue heading north on Illinois, turn right on 20th, and head back to the KT line stop at 20th and 3rd and your beginning.

Further Rambling

The Museum of Craft and Design (MCD), at No. 2569 3rd, is open to the public. Exhibits at the MCD change regularly, admission is free to members, and the new museum space provides public programming and art space for children to create their own crafts and designs.

The MUNI Woods Division, at No. 1001 22nd, which you pass when you walk back on Tennessee, is worth a quick peek. MUNI restores and refabricates cable cars as needed, and other historic fleet cars rely on this workshop for craftsman-style upkeep.

If the hills beyond Interstate 280 entice you, you could link this walk to Walk 22, Potrero Hill, by walking 12 blocks west on 20th, then turning left at De Haro.

You can also connect Walk 29 (The Blue Greenway) to this walk, especially if you'd like to take it in reverse. King St. is four stops away from Mariposa going inbound on the KT line; you can disembark there.

An Informal Bibliography

Adah has shared her books and research with me, and I have referenced many of the same titles she has, plus a few more. One of my favorites of the books that Adah has given me is Doris Muscatine's *Old San Francisco: The Biography of a City from Early Days to the Earthquake* (New York City: G. P. Putnam's Sons, 1975). I enjoy her writing as well as her scholarship and recommend it without reservation.

Also on my shelves is David Myrick's now out-of-print *San Francisco's Telegraph Hill* (Berkeley: Howell-North Books, 1972). It's a priceless history with archival photographs.

Trustworthy reference books to have on hand are: Gladys Hansen's *San Francisco Almanac* (San Francisco: Chronicle Books, 1995); Judith Lynch Waldhorn and Sally Woodbridge's *Victoria's Legacy: Tours of San Francisco Bay Area Architecture* (San Francisco: 101 Productions, 1978); William Kostura's *Russian Hill: The Summit, 1853–1906* (San Francisco: Aerie Publications, 1997); Amy Meyer's *New Guardians for the Golden Gate* (Berkeley: University of California Press, 2006), a beautifully told story of the 30-year effort of dedicated citizens to save the land that became Golden Gate National Recreation Area; and Doris Sloan's *Geology of the San Francisco Bay Region* (Berkeley: University of California Press, 2006).

When writing the St. Francis Wood walk, I found both the following sources invaluable: Mark A. Wilson's "Mason-McDuffie and the Creation of St. Francis Wood," published in *The Argonaut: Journal of the San Francisco Historical Society* (Fall 1997) and Jake Sigg's "New Zealand Christmas Tree," a pamphlet published by Friends of the Urban Forest in August–September 2006.

Randolph Delehanty's *Walks and Tours in the Golden Gate City* (San Francisco: The Dial Press, 1980) is an enlightening, opinionated commentary on the architecture throughout the city.

Appendix

List of Stairways

There is no such thing as a *complete* anything, but with 671 stairways, this list is rather comprehensive. We have listed all the public stairways *except* stairways that go up to a school, stairways that access private property, and stairways so decrepit that they are a danger to traverse. We have marked (with an asterisk, *) stairways in problematic neighborhoods. Long stairways that streets interrupt are counted as one stairway. Multiple stairways in parks have been listed as one.

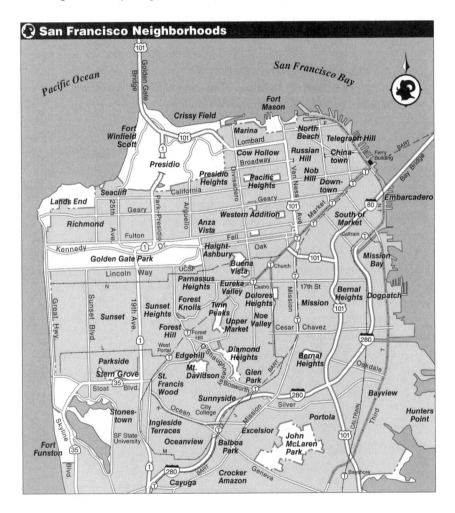

No single factor can sum up the character of a stairway. It may be 100 steps but easy (Diamond and 22nd St.) or 30 steps and difficult (Collingwood St.). We have charming stairways (Pemberton) and we have utilitarian stairways (Stonestown). We have elegant concrete stairways (Alta Plaza Park) and we have wood and concrete stairways (Joy). We have stairways bordered by trees, shrubs, flowers, stones, broken glass, railings, Victorian houses, and lean-tos.

Stairways are difficult to push into categories—it seems easier to classify neighborhoods than stairways. Forest Hill and Forest Knolls are unusual in settings and stairways. Golden Gate Heights and Noe Valley have well-designed networks of stairways and retaining walls. Diamond Heights has a series of very long stairways. Telegraph Hill and Russian Hill have alleys, stairways, and many houses without street access. Living along the Filbert and Greenwich Stairways in the Telegraph Hill area is an incentive to purchase lightweight furniture like futons. East Bernal Heights has become a forest of stairways, and several intersect community gardens.

Above all, this is a participatory book. The fun is in walking, discovering your own variations, and having conversations with neighborhood residents. The exhilarating views are just another bonus of this extraordinary city.

Ratings

Ratings are based on what resonated most during a walk: steepness, length, location, elevation, or beauty—and any combination of these attributes. The slash (/) stands for the word "between."

5 The Scheherazade category. These stairways surprise the walker. Elegant or rustic, short or long, they exhibit variety, stir the imagination, and delight the senses.

4 Impressive qualities with minor shortcomings; one outstanding aspect or extremely attractive section.

3 Little known but deserving of wider recognition because of the environs, human-made or natural. Neighborhood is generally very attractive.

2 Intrinsic to neighborhood history and ambiance. Well trodden. Functional. In most cases, the architectural context rates considerably higher than the stairway itself, or the view may be worth the visit.

1 It may be so boring that you'll fall asleep on the first landing.

* Worth visiting if it were located in a safe neighborhood; only for the knowledgeable resident, the wary aficionado.

ANZA VISTA

This neighborhood surrounding the University of San Francisco complex includes small, well-kept homes from the 1950s and the Victorian era.

RATING

2 Arbol Lane/Anza Vista & Turk. Good everyday route.

2 Arguella/Anza & Edward, into Rossi Recreation Center. Large granite planter bowls at entrance of two granite stairways.

3 Blake/Geary & Euclid, into Laurel Hill Playground. In Laurel Heights.

2 Cook/Geary & Euclid. In Laurel Heights. View of Lone Mtn.

2 Dicha Alley/Lupine & Wood. Useful and used.

2 Ewing at Nos. 196–200 to Anza, near Collins. Ewing Court was a baseball field at one time. Clever.

4 Lone Mtn., from No. 401 Parker to Beaumont to Stanyan to Rossi. Long twitton trees, church spires, views of Angel Island and west; nice series of Victorians on McAllister off Parker.

2 O'Farrell & Lyon. Rounding a corner.

1 Sonora Lane/Terra Vista & O'Farrell at No. 90 Terra Vista.

BALBOA PARK

American Indian street names abound in this neighborhood. It has underground waterways, a creek, and the old Cayuga Lake.

RATING

2 Alemany, near Rousseau to Mission.

2 Balboa Park. San Jose, near Ocean, into park.

2 Geneva, near Ocean. Skyway to City College; stairways midspan to MUNI Metro.

1 Mission at Trumbull to Alemany.

2 Naglee/Alemany & Cayuga.

2 Oneida/Alemany & Cayuga.

1 Restani/Restani Way & No. 718 Geneva.

BART AND MUNI METRO STATIONS

RATING

2 Balboa Park BART-Muni Metro Station at Geneva & San Jose, down into station.

2 Civic Center BART Station at 8th & Market, down into station.

1 Embarcadero BART-Muni Metro Station at Embarcadero/Market, down into station.

2 Forest Hill MUNI Metro Station at Laguna Honda, near Dewey, inside station.

3 Glen Park BART Station at Diamond/Bosworth & Monterey, down into station.

2 Glen Park BART Station at Monterey at Diamond.

2 Market. Castro MUNI Metro Station at Castro & Market, down into station.

3 Market. Church at Market, down into MUNI Metro Station.

3 Mission. 16th St. BART Station at Mission, down into station.

3 Mission. 24th St. BART Station at Mission, down into station.

3 Montgomery BART-Muni Metro Station at Montgomery & Market, down into station.

4 Powell BART-Muni Metro Station at Powell & Market, down into station.

2 Van Ness MUNI Metro Station at Van Ness & Market, down into station.

2 West Portal MUNI Metro Station at West Portal & Santa Clara, down into station.

BAYVIEW

This neighborhood has some historic buildings.

RATING

* Bayview Park.
* Gilroy & Jamestown.
* Hawes & Innes.
* Hilltop Park. Lillian at Beatrice, up to park.
* Hilltop Park. LaSalle at Osceola, up to park.
* Key/3rd St. & Bayview Park entrance.
* Key at Jennings.
* Lane to No. 1501 Lower LaSalle.
* LaSalle to Health Center/Osceola & Garlington Court.
* LaSalle & Osceola to Health Center.
* LaSalle–Upper LaSalle to Lindsay Circle.
* Mini Park at Lillian & Rosie Lee Lane.
* Quesada/Newhall & 3rd St.
* Quesada–Upper Quesada to Lower Quesada, near Newhall.
* Revere/Newhall & 3rd St. Sidewalk stairway.
* Thornton/3rd St. & Latona.

BERNAL HEIGHTS

A neighborhood mix of professionals, blue-collar workers, and artists. Most stairways have adjoining gardens.

RATING

4 Andover/Powhattan & Bernal Heights Park.

1   Appleton/San Jose & Mission.

2   Aztec/Aztec & Shotwell.

3   Banks/Chapman & Powhattan.

2   Bernal Heights Park. Coso, near Bonview, into park.

3   Bernal Heights Park. Across street from 39 Ellsworth into park.

2   Bernal Heights Park. End of Esmeralda Stwy. up to trail and into park.

3   Bessie/Bessie & Mirabel at Shotwell.

4   Brewster/Brewster at Costa & Upper Brewster & Rutledge.

2   Bronte, uphill from Cortland, south.

1   Bronte/Tompkins & Jarboe.

3   Chapman to Powhattan at Nevada.

2   Coso/Prospect & Winfield.

2   Cuvier/San Jose & Bosworth.

3   Esmeralda/Brewster & Franconia.

5   Esmeralda/Coleridge & Bernal Heights Park.

1   Esmeralda-Upper Esmeralda to Lower Esmeralda at Peralta.

4   Eugenia/Prospect & Winfield.

1   Eve Stwy./Upper & Lower Holladay at Wright & Peralta.

3   Fair Stwy./Coleridge & Prospect.

3   Faith/Brewster & Holladay.

4   Franconia/Franconia & Brewster Stwy.

3   Franconia/Montcalm & Rutledge.

3   Franconia/Mullen & Montcalm.

3   Franconia/Mullen & Peralta.

4   Gates/Bernal Heights Blvd. & Powhattan.

3   Harrison/Ripley & Norwich.

1   Highland to San Jose.

4   Holladay/Peralta & Bayshore.

2   Holly Park. Across from Junipero Serra School at Holly Park Circle.

2   Holly Park. Boscana at Holly Park Circle, into park.

2   Holly Park. East side up from Highland, in park.

2   Holly Park. Highland at Holly Park Circle, into park.

2   Holly Park. Murray at Holly Park Circle, into park.

5   Joy/Holladay & Brewster.

3   Kingston/Coleridge & Prospect.

2   Manchester at end of street below Bernal Heights Park.

3   Mayflower/Holladay & Franconia.

3 Mayflower/Bradford & Carver.

5 Mirabel at No. 11 to Percita.

2 Montcalm/Wright & Peralta.

3 Montezuma at Coso to Mirabel.

3 Moultrie/Bernal Heights Blvd. & Powhattan.

2 Mullen Stwy., next to No. 146, near Franconia.

4 Ogden/Nevada & Prentiss.

2 Peralta Point Open Space/Montcalm & Mullen.

2 Peralta/Rutledge & Montcalm.

4 Peralta/Samoset & Rutledge.

2 Powhattan/Gates & Ellsworth.

4 Prentiss/Bernal Heights Blvd. & Powhattan.

2 Prospect/Cortland & Santa Maria.

1 Richland to San Jose.

3 Rosenkrantz/Bernal Heights Blvd. & Bernal Heights Blvd. at Powhattan.

4 Rutledge/Holladay, Mullen, Brewster, & Wolf Patch Community Garden.

3 Tompkins/Putnam & Nevada.

3 Virginia/Eugenia & Winfield.

BUENA VISTA (CORONA HEIGHTS)

An old neighborhood with large mansions and converted flats.

RATING

3 Alpine/Waller & Duboce.

4 Buena Vista East. Baker & Haight, into Buena Vista Park.

2 Buena Vista East. At Buena Vista Blvd. Nos. 75–101, 95, 135, 351, 437, into Buena Vista Park.

5 Buena Vista East. Buena Vista Blvd. at Nos. 355–399, into Buena Vista Park.

5 Buena Vista East. Buena Vista Terrace & Duboce, into Buena Vista Park.

3 Buena Vista East. Park Hill, into Buena Vista Park.

4 Buena Vista East. Waller/Broderick & Buena Vista at No. 101.

5 Buena Vista East. Waller/Broderick, into Buena Vista Park.

5 Buena Vista East & Buena Vista West at Upper Terrace.

2 Buena Vista West. Buena Vista Blvd. Nos. 555 & 737, into Buena Vista Park.

2 Buena Vista West. Central, into Buena Vista Park.

3 Buena Vista West. Frederick, into Buena Vista Park.

4 Buena Vista West. Haight/Central & Lyon, into Buena Vista Park. Lovely.

4 Buena Vista West. Java, into Buena Vista Park.

3 Buena Vista West. Lyon & Haight, into Buena Vista Park.

4 Buena Vista West. Welland Lathrop Memorial Walk, into Buena Vista Park, across from No. 547 Buena Vista West.

3 Buena Vista Park.

4 Corona Heights Park.

3 DeForest/Beaver & Flint.

3 Duboce/Castro & Divisadero.

3 Duboce/Divisadero & Alpine.

4 Henry Stwy./No. 473 Roosevelt & Castro.

CHINATOWN

A special combination of sounds, smells, and colors.

RATING

5 California/opposite No. 660, into St. Mary's Square.

2 Grant & Bush Stwy. & Chinatown Gate.

5 Portsmouth Square. Clay/Kearny & Walter Lum Pl.

5 Portsmouth Square. Interior of square toward Kearny.

5 Portsmouth Square. Kearny & Clay.

5 Portsmouth Square. Kearny & Washington.

5 Portsmouth Square. Walter Lum Pl./Clay & Washington.

5 Portsmouth Square. Washington & Walter Lum Pl.

DIAMOND HEIGHTS

A neighborhood of views, hills, and canyons.

RATING

4 Coralino/No. 289 Amber to No. 92 Cameo.

2 Diamond Heights Blvd. & No. 5411, into Walter Haas Park.

5 Glen Canyon Park to George Christopher Park, Crags Court, and Berkeley Way.

4 Gold Mine & No. 98 to Douglass & No. 681 28th St.

5 Gold Mine at No. 160/Ora & Jade (Opalo).

5 Onique/No. 101 Berkeley, No. 289 Berkeley, No. 400 Gold Mine & No. 243 Topaz.

2 Safira Lane/27th St. at No. 881 & Diamond Heights Blvd. at Nos. 5173 & 5147, adjoining Douglass Playground.

3 Turquoise/No. 48 & No. 52.

DOGPATCH

1 Tennessee/No. 1108 & No. 1110

DOLORES HEIGHTS

A lovely, hilly neighborhood in the Mission District.

RATING

2 Cumberland/Church & Dolores Park.

5 Cumberland/Noe No. 670 & Sanchez.

4 Cumberland/Sanchez & Church.

3 Dolores Park.

3 Dolores Park. 19th St./Church & Dolores Park, over MUNI Metro tracks.

2 Hancock/Church & Dolores Park.

5 Liberty/Noe & Rayburn.

4 Liberty/Sanchez & Church.

2 Sanchez/Cumberland & Sanchez Stwy.

5 Sanchez/Liberty & 21st St.

4 Sanchez/19th St. & Cumberland.

5 20th St. & Noe.

5 20th St. & Sanchez.

3 21st St./Castro & Collingwood.

3 22nd St./Castro & Collingwood.

4 22nd St./Church & Vicksburg.

4 22nd St./Diamond & Collingwood.

DOWNTOWN

A neighborhood subject to significant changes.

RATING

2 Stockton Tunnel/Sutter & Bush and Sacramento & California.

3 Union Square. Multiple stairways on Post, Stockton, & Geary/Stockton & Powell and Geary & Post.

4 Union Square. Powell & Geary, into square.

3 Union Square. Powell & Post, into square.

4 Union Square. Stockton & Geary, into square.

3 Union Square. Stockton & Post, into square.

EDGEHILL

The steepness of the hill limits the number of homes on this street, which winds up to the summit.

RATING

3   Dorchester to Kensington. Crosses Allston & Granville.

3   Edgehill Open Space.

2   Garcia/Edgehill Way & Idora, connecting Upper and Lower Garcia.

2   Garcia/Vasquez & Edgehill Way, connecting Upper and Lower Garcia.

2   Idora/Garcia & Laguna Honda, connecting Upper and Lower Idora.

1   Lennox, opposite No. 146.

5   Pacheco/Merced & Vasquez.

3   Ulloa/Kensington & Waithman.

2   Ulloa at Waithman.

2   West Portal Drive & No. 21.

EMBARCADERO

Area has been revitalized. The Farmers' Market at the Ferry Building is one of the most popular attractions in the city.

RATING

5   Commercial/Sansome & No. 1 Embarcadero Center.

2   Embarcadero Center.

2   Ferry Building at North End Plaza.

3   Justin Herman Plaza at end of Market & Embarcadero.

4   Maritime Plaza/Washington/Clay/Battery/Front & Davis.

2   Pacific/Battery & Sansome, into Masto Plaza.

EUREKA VALLEY

This neighborhood has a community organization that has been active since 1881, a large gay population, fine Victorians, beautiful gardens, and the Castro (a movie palace built in 1922).

RATING

1   Acme Alley/Corwin No. 95 & Grand View.

3   Caselli/Clayton & Market.

3   Clover Lane/No. 101 Caselli & No. 4612 19th St. Cross alley and continue up.

2   Dixie/No. 3801 Market & No. 285 Grand View near Alvarado.

4   Douglass at Corwin.

3   Douglass at No. 414/Corwin & Romain.

3 Douglass at Romain.

1 Douglass at 19th St.

4 Douglass/20th St. & Corwin.

1 Douglass at 24th St., into Noe Valley Park.

2 Grand View to Market, near Grand View Terrace.

3 Grand View to Stanton at Market.

3 Mono/Market & Eagle, with a ramp to Caselli.

3 19th St. at No. 4612 to Kite Hill.

2 Prosper/16th St. & Pond.

3 Seward at Douglass & No. 31 Seward.

2 Seward at No. 30.

4 Short/Market & Yukon.

1 Upper Market Walkway/Glendale & Romain.

3 Yukon/Eagle & Short.

EXCELSIOR (McLAREN PARK)

A stable neighborhood of diverse ethnic groups. Stairways reminiscent of the everyday kind of European towns.

RATING

2 Athens/Avalon & Peru.

2 Crocker-Amazon Park. Geneva, opposite No. 1572, into park.

3 Crocker-Amazon Park. Prague, near Russia, into park.

2 Crocker-Amazon Playground Skate Park to McLaren Park.

2 Kenney Alley at No. 646 London to Mission.

1 Lisbon/Russia & France.

3 McLaren Park. Ervine at Wilde.

2 McLaren Park. Excelsior at No. 1021, near Munich, into park.

2 McLaren Park. LaGrande & Brazil, into park.

2 McLaren Park. On the path/Lake McNab & Shelley Dr.

2 McLaren Park. On the path/Shelley Lake & Shelley Dr.

3 McLaren Park. Prague at Brazil, into park.

2 McLaren Park. Prague at Excelsior, into park.

2 McLaren Park. University at Woolsey, into park.

2 McLaren Park. Yale, into park.

4 Munich/Ina & Excelsior.

4 Peru/Athens & Valmar.

2 Sunglow Lane/Gladstone & Silver at Oxford.

FOREST HILL

The city has accepted responsibility for maintaining the nonregulation streets of this neighborhood.

RATING

4   Alton/Lower Pacheco to No. 399 Upper Pacheco, continuing to No. 60 Sotelo.

4   Alton/No. 60 Ventura to No. 70 Alton & No. 400 Lower Pacheco.

4   Castenada at No. 140 to Pacheco at No. 334.

2   Castenada, opposite No. 249.

2   Dorantes & Magellan.

2   Dorantes & San Marcos.

5   8th Ave. at No. 1998 to No. 20 Ventura.

2   Forest Hill MUNI Metro Station, to Magellan.

5   Montalvo/Castenada at No. 376 to San Marcos to 9th Ave. to Mendosa.

2   Murphy Playground/9th Ave. & 8th Ave., near Pacheco.

5   Pacheco/Magellan & No. 249 Castenada.

2   Pacheco–Upper Pacheco at No. 364 to Lower Pacheco.

5   Santa Rita at No. 60 to Upper and Lower San Marcos.

2   12th Ave. (at end) to Dorantes.

FOREST KNOLLS

A neighborhood heavily forested with eucalyptus.

RATING

4   Ashwood Lane/Clarendon & Warren at No. 101.

4   Blairwood Lane/No. 113 Warren & No. 95 & No. 101 Crestmont.

2   Forest Knolls Stwy. at No. 191 Forest Knolls Drive, in cul-de-sac, down to school playground.

3   Glenhaven Lane/Oak Park & No. 191 Christopher.

5   Oakhurst Lane/Warren & Crestmont.

FORT FUNSTON

Part of Golden Gate National Recreation Area; off CA Hwy. 35, south of the zoo.

RATING

4   Horsetail Stwy., left of parking lot.

2   John Muir Drive at Skyline, on path to Fort Funston.

1   Multiple stairways at gunnery and battery sites in Fort Funston.

FORT MASON

Magnificent example of conversion from military fort to part of the Golden Gate National Recreation Area.

RATING

2 Alcatraz Island.

2 Aquatic Park Promenade & Upper Railroad-Tie Walkway/Polk & Van Ness.

4 Fort Mason. Black Point Battery to Aquatic Park.

2 Fort Mason. Black Point Battery to top of wall.

3 Fort Mason. Black Point Gunnery behind San Francisco International Youth Hostel.

2 Fort Mason. Community Garden.

3 Fort Mason. End of Franklin to Black Point Battery & picnic area.

3 Fort Mason. Great Meadow & Building E at Pier 3.

3 Fort Mason. Great Meadow & San Francisco International Youth Center near Bufano Peace sculpture.

4 Jefferson/Beach, Hyde & Larkin. Amphitheater in Victoria Park.

FORT WINFIELD SCOTT

A fort within the Presidio with beautiful rock walls, stairs, and vegetation.

RATING

5 Batteries to Bluffs/Langdon & Marshall Beach & Baker Beach.

4 Kobbe, opposite No. 1324 to tennis practice area.

4 Kobbe, opposite No. 1328 to tennis courts.

4 Kobbe, opposite No. 1330, at parking area to recreation hall.

1 Multiple stairways at gunnery and battery sites in Fort Scott.

3 Native Plant Garden, to upper nursery.

2 Ruckman/Appleton & Ralston. Left sidewalk stairway.

2 Tennis courts: Multiple stairways into and around.

4 Wool Court & Upton, opposite No. 1337 Pope sign to tennis courts parking lot.

5 Wool Court & Upton intersection.

GLEN PARK

Cows roamed the meadowland in this neighborhood in the 1880s.

RATING

3 Amatista Lane/Bemis, near Miguel to Everson.

2 Bemis, Nos. 130 & 134 at Mateo.

3 Billy Goat Hill.

2   Burnside at Bosworth, across from No. 1035 Bosworth.

2   Chilton at Bosworth, across from No. 907 Bosworth.

2   Diamond & Moffit.

2   Glen Canyon Park. Bosworth at No. 1231, into park.

3   Glen Canyon Park. Elk at Sussex, into park.

3   Glen Canyon Park to George Christopher Park, Crags Court, Berkeley Way.

2   Glen Park Village Garden. Diamond at No. 2783, into garden.

2   Hamerton/Bosworth & Mangels.

5   Harry Stwy. at No. 190 Beacon to Laidley.

1   Penny Lane/Diamond at Castro.

1   Roanoke/San Jose & Arlington.

2   St. Mary's/San Jose & Arlington at No. 439.

GOLDEN GATE HEIGHTS

Carl Larsen, from Denmark, deeded this acreage to the city in 1928.

RATING

4   Aerial Way/14th Ave. & Funston.

3   Aerial Way/No. 475 Ortega & No. 801 Pacheco.

2   Aloha & Lomita.

5   Cascade Walk/Ortega, Pacheco, & Funston.

2   8th Ave./Moraga & Lawton.

2   Fanning & 14th Ave.

2   Fanning & 15th Ave.

4   15th Ave./Kirkham & Lawton.

1   15th Ave., near Fanning & Quintara.

2   15th Ave., near Moraga to Upper 15th.

2   Golden Gate Heights Park. Radio & 12th Ave.

5   Golden Gate Heights Park. 12th Ave. & Cragmont, into park to tennis courts.

3   Golden Gate Heights Park. 12th Ave. at playground, to tennis courts.

3   Grand View Park.

4   Grand View Park. 14th Ave. to the top of park.

4   Grand View Park. Upper 15th Ave. to the top of park.

4   Mandalay Lane/No. 2001 14th Ave. & 15th Ave. & Pacheco.

5   Moraga/15th & 16th Aves.

5   Moraga/Funston & top of Grand View Park.

4 Mount/No. 1795 14th Ave. & No. 1798 15th Ave.

2 9th Ave./Lawton & Moraga.

4 Noriega to 15th Ave. & Sheldon Terrace.

4 Oriole Way/Pacheco & Cragmont.

4 Ortega Way/14th Ave. & No. 1894 15th Ave.

4 Pacheco & 12th Ave.

2 Pacheco & 14th Ave.

4 Pacheco/14th & 15th Ave.

3 Pacheco & 16th Ave.

4 Quintara at No. 500/14th and 15th Aves.

3 Quintara & 16th Ave.

5 Selma Way/No. 477 Noriega & No. 564 Ortega.

5 16th Ave./Kirkham & Lawton.

3 16th Ave./Pacheco & Quintara.

GOLDEN GATE PARK

Stairs are still being built here.

RATING

5 AIDS Memorial.

3 Anglers Lodge, off JFK Drive, opposite buffalo paddock.

2 Big recreation area. Street to tennis courts.

3 Botanical Garden and Arboretum/Martin Luther King Drive & 9th Ave.

2 Children's Playground.

3 Children's Playground to Kezar Court.

3 Conservatory of Flowers. Right side, east to Dahlia Gardens.

4 Conservatory of Flowers. To walkway and front entrance from lawn area.

3 Fulton at Arguello.

2 Fulton at 6th Ave.

3 Fulton at 10th Ave.

3 Horseshoe Court near Conservatory Drive East & Arguello.

2 Japanese Tea Garden/Back of garden & east side of Stow Lake.

3 JFK Drive: Down to Chain of Lakes, north side.

3 JFK Drive: Intersection of Bernice Rogers Way & JFK Drive.

1 JFK Drive: Up to restrooms past buffalo paddock.

2 Lincoln at 7th Ave., into Golden Gate Park.

2 Martin Luther King Drive. Baseball court at 7th Ave.

2   Martin Luther King Drive. Murphy Windmill & Great Highway.

2   Martin Luther King Drive. Street to Stow Lake.

2   Martin Luther King Drive. West at 19th Ave.

4   Stanyan/Haight & Waller, into Golden Gate Park.

3   Stow Lake. Huntington Falls/Stow Lake Shore and top of Strawberry Hill.

5   Stow Lake. Strawberry Hill/Stow Lake Shore and top of hill at bridge.

2   Stow Lake. To Strawberry Hill/Chinese Pavilion & Falls Stairway.

HAIGHT-ASHBURY

Deliberate remnants of the 1960s counterculture in Lower Haight. Upper Haight is a stable community of professionals and middle-class families. Beautiful Victorians.

RATING

2   Clayton/Frederick & Carl.

5   Frederick & Carl/Arguello & Willard, opposite Kezar Stadium. Parkview Commons.

2   Frederick at Willard.

INGLESIDE TERRACE

Well-planned community west of Twin Peaks and near San Francisco State University with curved streets. Developed by Joseph Leonard around 1913. Famous for its large sundial and early racetrack.

RATING

2   Alemany & Head St., near Palmetto.

2   Alemany, opposite Victoria.

3   San Leandro at No. 344/Moncado & Ocean.

2   Shakespeare/Shakespeare & DeLong.

2   Worcester, near Alemany.

3   Wyton/19th Ave. & Junipero Serra.

LANDS END

Great area for ocean breezes and beaches.

RATING

3   Coastal Trail to El Camino del Mar Trail, just below the VA Medical Center.

4   Coastal Trail.

3   Multiple stairways connecting trails in the area.

2   Eagle's Point at El Camino del Mar.

3   El Camino del Mar Trail/back of Palace of Legion of Honor & USS *San Francisco Naval Memorial*.

5 Mile Rock Stwy./Coastal Trail & Mile Rock Beach.

5 Sutro Baths Stwy./Merrie Way parking lot & Sutro Baths.

4 USS *San Francisco Naval Memorial* Stwy./48th Ave. & El Camino del Mar to the Coastal Trail.

MARINA

Development of this neighborhood was given impetus from the 1915 Panama-Pacific International Exposition.

RATING

2 Bay St./Webster & Buchanan, into George Moscone Recreation Center.

2 Crissy Field entrance to St. Francis Yacht Club at Lyon, to benches and to water.

3 Wave Organ at end of jetty by Golden Gate Yacht Club, around structure and down to water.

MISSION

One of the largest districts in San Francisco. Divided into more than a dozen subneighborhoods.

RATING

3 Franklin Square. Bryant at 16th St., into square.

3 Franklin Square. Bryant at 17th St., into square.

3 Franklin Square. 17th St./Bryant & Potrero, into square.

1 Garfield Square. Harrison at 25th & 26th Sts., into square.

1 Garfield Square. Harrison/25th & 26th Sts., into square.

1 Garfield Square. Treat at 26th St., into square.

2 25th St./Fair Oaks & Dolores.

MT. DAVIDSON

A neighborhood circling the highest elevation in San Francisco (938 feet). The cross and the surrounding plateau are now privately owned. Be cautious. Fog can make the stairways wet.

RATING

2 Acova Alley/No. 219 Bella Vista Way at 550 Myra, opposite Dorcas Way.

3 Burlwood & Los Palmos.

3 Casitas at Cresta Vista.

2 Chaves & Del Sur.

2 Globe Alley at No. 96 Cresta Vista to Hazelwood, near Los Palmos.

2 Hazelwood & Los Palmos.

2   Lulu Alley/Los Palmos & No. 450 to No. 500 Melrose.

3   Malta/Upper Malta No. 11 and Lower Malta No. 50.

3   Mangels/Brentwood & Melrose.

2   Marietta–Upper Marietta at No. 466 to Lower Marietta.

2   Melrose at Mangels & Ridgewood.

2   Miraloma at No. 2 to Portola.

4   Mt. Davidson. Juanita Way at No. 275 Juanita, near Marne.

3   Mt. Davidson. Rockdale Drive, next to Nos. 919 and 925.

2   Mt. Davidson & St. Croix Road.

3   Mt. Davidson Summit (three trails).

4   Mt. Davidson Summit (two trails).

4   Mt. Davidson Summit. East Ridge Trail and Sherwood Trail at summit.

2   Vista Verde Court at Stillings.

3   Yerba Buena, near Maywood, to Miraloma.

3   Yerba Buena to Upper Yerba Buena at Ravenswood.

NOB HILL

A famous neighborhood well-known to tourists.

RATING

2   Clay to Washington, opposite No. 1171 Clay.

4   Grace Cathedral at California & Taylor.

3   Huntington Park. California at Taylor & Cushman Alley, into park.

3   Huntington Park. Sacramento at Taylor & Cushman Alley, into park.

3   Huntington Park. Taylor/California & Sacramento, into park.

4   Joice Alley at Pine to Sacramento/Powell & Stockton.

2   Mason at California.

2   Phoenix, opposite No. 1154 Pacific/Taylor & Jones.

2   Priest, opposite No. 1350 Washington.

2   Reed, opposite No. 1370 Washington.

3   Taylor/Pine & California.

NOE VALLEY

An authentic neighborhood.

RATING

3   Castro/Day & No. 500 30th St.

4   Castro/28th St. & Duncan.

3   Cesar Chavez/Castro at No. 4220 & Diamond.

3   Cuesta Court to Grand View at No. 601, near 24th St.

4 Cuesta Court/Portola & Corbett.

3 Day at No. 493, up to No. 2350 Castro.

2 Duncan/Noe toward Sanchez.

4 Elizabeth/Hoffman & Grand View.

2 Noe/Cesar Chavez & 27th St.

3 27th St. at Castro & Newberg.

3 27th St./Castro & Noe, from cul-de-sac at end of 27th St. to Noe.

2 Valley/Castro to Noe.

3 Valley/Diamond & Castro.

NORTH BEACH

A neighborhood in transition from predominantly Italian settlers to Chinese.

RATING

4 Kearny/Vallejo & Broadway.

2 Powell at Filbert, into Washington Square Playground.

2 Romolo/Vallejo & Fresno, west of Kearny.

3 Tuscany at Lombard/Stockton & Powell.

2 Wayne at Pacific/Mason & Powell.

PACIFIC HEIGHTS

A neighborhood that has maintained its standards in architecture and appearance. Enviable views and private schools.

RATING

1 Allyne Park at Green & Gough.

3 Alta Plaza.

5 Alta Plaza. Pierce at Clay, into park.

3 Alta Plaza. Pierce at Jackson, into park.

5 Alta Plaza. Scott/Clay & Washington, into park.

5 Alta Plaza. Steiner/Clay & Washington, into park.

5 Alta Plaza. Steiner at Washington, into park.

2 Baker/Green & Vallejo.

5 Baker/Vallejo & Broadway.

4 Broderick/Broadway & Vallejo.

5 Fillmore/Broadway & Green.

4 Green/Scott & Pierce.

3 Lafayette Park. Gough at Clay, into park, connecting on path to tennis courts.

3 Lafayette Park. Gough at Sacramento, into park.

3 Lafayette Park. Gough at Washington, into park.

2 Lafayette Park. Interior of the park.

1 Lafayette Park. Laguna at Sacramento, into park.

3 Lafayette Park. Laguna at Washington, into park.

5 Lyon/Green & Vallejo & Broadway.

4 Normandie Terrace at Vallejo.

3 Octavia/Washington & Jackson.

1 Vallejo at Lyon.

3 Vallejo/Scott & Pierce.

3 Webster/Broadway & Vallejo.

PARKSIDE

A community of pluses and minuses. From sand dunes and fog to flowers and ethnic diversity.

RATING

2 Judah/LaPlaya & Great Highway.

2 McCoppin Square. 22nd Ave., near Taraval.

2 Stern Grove. 19th Ave. & Sloat.

PARNASSUS HEIGHTS

Home of the University of California (UC) Medical School, with Sutro Forest as the background.

RATING

2 Belgrave, at end of street, to Tank Hill.

1 Belgrave, near Stanyan, into interior Park Belt.

3 Farnsworth/Edgewood & Willard.

3 Kirkham at 4th Ave., up to 1550 5th Ave., behind UC Medical School.

3 Stanyan, near No. 1289/Belgrave & 17th St. Stairways on both sides of street.

PORTOLA

A neighborhood showing strains.

RATING

2 Campus Lane/Princeton & Burrows.

3 Dwight/Goettingen & Hamilton.

3 Goettingen & Dwight.

POTRERO HILL

Beautiful weather and views.

RATING

3 Carolina/19th & 20th Sts.

3 Carolina at Southern Heights.

1 Connecticut (end), up to Arkansas at 22nd St. Stwy.

4 Kansas/22nd & 21st Sts., from No. 980 to No. 965 Kansas.

2 Mariposa/Utah & Potrero.

2-3 McKinley Square.

4 McKinley Square Playground. San Bruno at 20th St., into square.

3 McKinley Square Playground. Vermont at 20th St., into square.

2 19th St./De Haro & Rhode Island.

2 24th St./Rhode Island & De Haro.

3 22nd St./ Wisconsin & Connecticut, into Potrero Hill Recreation Center.

2 22nd St./Kansas & Rhode Island.

3 23rd St./Lower Carolina & Upper Carolina.

3 23rd St./Carolina & Wisconsin.

4 Vermont/20th St. to 22nd St.

PRESIDIO

Founded in 1776 by the Spanish under Jose Joaquin Moraga and Juan Bautista de Anza. Obtain a map of the area at the Visitors' Center.

RATING

2 Baker Beach, up to Baker Beach Road.

3 Baker Beach Stwy. Lincoln Blvd./Pershing Drive & Kobbe Ave. to Baker Beach.

3 Coastal Trail/Golden Gate Bridge & Fort Point.

2 Coastal Trail just east of Golden Gate Bride.

3-4 Coastal Trail just east of Golden Gate Bridge.

5 Connector stairways. Between Park Blvd. & Cemetery Overlook; between Lincoln Blvd. & Immigrant Overlook & Rob Hill Campground.

2 8th Ave./Lake & Mountain Lake Park.

2 Golden Gate Bridge.

4 Letterman Digital Arts Center. Gorgas Gate at Gorgas & Lyon.

4 Letterman Digital Arts Center. Park Garden/Chestnut & Francisco.

2 Lincoln Blvd. at Hoffman.

3 MacArthur Ave., to end at El Polin Spring.

3   Moraga/Funston & Barnard.

1   Multiple stairways at gunnery and battery sites in the Presidio.

3   Multiple stairways. Simonds Loop, Gibbon Ct., Infantry Terrace, and Amatury Loop.

2   Presidio Blvd. at Nos. 548–550, near MacArthur Ave./Lombard & Lincoln Blvd.

2   12th Ave. at playground into Mountain Lake Park.

1   Young & Lincoln.

1   Young to Presidio Post, behind Crissy Field Center.

RICHMOND

Known as the "sand waste" area in early days of San Francisco.
RATING

4   Balboa/No. 641 48th Ave. & LaPlaya.

5   California/32nd Ave. & golf course, to Lincoln Park.

2   Clement/43rd and 44th Aves. up to VA Medical Center.

2   48th Ave. & Balboa.

2   Great Hwy./Balboa & Sloat.

4   Lake/El Camino del Mar to 30th Ave.

5   Sutro Heights Park at 48th Ave./Point Lobos Ave. & Anza.

4   3rd Ave. Nos. 1–11 at Lake.

RUSSIAN HILL

Graves of Russians buried on the hill account for the neighborhood name.
RATING

2   Broadway/Jones and Taylor.

1   Broadway Tunnel West Mini Park/Cyrus & Hyde.

1   Broadway Tunnel East Mini Park/Himmelman Place at Broadway.

5   Chestnut/Polk & Larkin.

3   Culebra Terrace/No. 1250 Lombard & Chestnut.

5   Filbert/Hyde & Leavenworth.

3   Florence/Broadway & Vallejo.

3   Francisco/Lower Leavenworth & Francisco.

5   Francisco/Upper Leavenworth & Hyde.

2   George Sterling Park at Larkin & Lombard.

4   Green/Jones & Taylor, next to No. 940 Green.

5   Greenwich/Hyde & Larkin.

5   Greenwich/Hyde & Leavenworth.

5   Greenwich (south side)/Leavenworth & Jones.

1 Hastings/Filbert & Union.

4 Havens/Leavenworth & Hyde, in cul-de-sac.

2 Himmelman Place to Salmon.

1 Houston/Jones & Columbus, next to 2430 Jones.

3 Hyde & Francisco.

5 Jones/Filbert & Union & Green.

3 Jones: Upper to Lower Jones at Vallejo.

3 Larkin/Chestnut & Francisco, beginning at No. 2745 Larkin.

4 Larkin/Francisco & Bay.

5 Lombard/Hyde & Leavenworth.

2/5 Macondray Lane/Leavenworth & Taylor.

3 Montclair Terrace/Lombard & Chestnut.

1 Redfield Alley.

3 Russian Hill Park at Bay/Hyde & Larkin.

5 Vallejo/Jones & Taylor.

5 Vallejo/Mason & Taylor.

2 Valparaiso/Filbert & Greenwich on Taylor.

ST. FRANCIS WOOD

One of the finest residential parks designed west of Twin Peaks. Developed by Mason & McDuffie between 1912 and 1918.

RATING

3 Junipero Serra to Santa Ana/Darian & Monterey.

3 Portola at Santa Clara.

3 St. Francis Blvd. at San Anselmo, Upper Fountain.

3 St. Francis Blvd. at Santa Ana, Lower Fountain.

2 San Anselmo & Santa Ana at Portola.

1 Stonestown Stwy./19th Ave. & Stonestown Center.

2 Terrace Drive at Terrace Walk Stwy.

2 Terrace Drive, opposite No. 141.

5 Terrace Walk/San Anselmo & Yerba Buena.

SEACLIFF

Beautiful ocean views and large homes. A hop and skip from Lands End hiking trails and the Palace of the Legion of Honor.

RATING

1 China Beach.

3 China Beach Road, opposite No. 455, from path to China Beach.

4 Seacliff.

4   Seacliff at No. 330.

2   Seacliff. North 25th Ave. in Seacliff, to Baker Beach.

4   Seacliff. 27th Ave./Seacliff & El Camino del Mar.

SOUTH OF MARKET

Once an early residential neighborhood—subsequently industrial, presently mixed. Changed to lofts; AT&T Park (home of the San Francisco Giants); Mission Bay campus of the University of California, San Francisco Medical Center; and condos.

RATING

3   Beale/Main & Fremont to Harrison, opposite No. 228.

3   Bryant/1st St. & Rincon.

*   Lansing/1st St. & Essex.

4   Yerba Buena Gardens/Mission & Howard, 3rd & 4th Sts.

3   Yerba Buena Lane at 757 Market to Mission/2nd & 3rd Sts.

SUNNYSIDE

A neighborhood worth exploring.

RATING

4   Detroit/Joost, Monterey, & Hearst.

2   Forester at Melrose, across from Sunnyside Playground.

5   Joost and Baden Mini Park/Nos. 242 & 250 Joost and Nos. 149 & 151 Mangels.

4   Melrose Stwy./Teresita to Mangels to Sunnyside Playground.

2   Monterey: Upper Monterey to Lower Monterey at Plymouth.

5   Next to No. 233 Joost, down to Monterey Blvd., via historic Sunnyside Conservatory.

TELEGRAPH HILL

Early photographs show stairways literally hanging over the cliffs of this historic neighborhood. Three new stairways leading to Coit Tower were built in 2005.

RATING

2   Bartol Alley at No. 379 Broadway to Vallejo.

3   Child/Lombard & Telegraph Place.

4   Coit Tower. Down to path (west side).

2   Coit Tower. Entrance (north side).

3   Coit Tower. Rear lawn area. Pioneer Park.

4 Coit Tower. Rear path to Telegraph Hill Blvd. (south side).

5 Filbert/Grant & Kearny, next to Garfield School.

3 Filbert/Kearny & Telegraph Hill Blvd.

5 Filbert/Telegraph Hill Blvd. & Montgomery & Sansome.

4 Francisco/Kearny & Grant.

2 Genoa Place/Filbert & Union.

4 Grant/Francisco & Chestnut.

4 Greenwich/Grant & Telegraph Hill Blvd.

5 Greenwich/Telegraph Hill Blvd. & Montgomery & Sansome.

3 Julius/Lombard & Whiting.

1 Krausgrill at Filbert, near Stockton.

5 Lombard at Telegraph Hill Blvd., near Kearny.

4 Montgomery/Green & Union.

3 Pardee Alley/Grant & Kramer.

2 San Antonio Place/Vallejo & Kearny.

3 Telegraph Hill Blvd. at Greenwich Stwy. (west side).

4 Union/Calhoun & east cliff of Telegraph Hill.

1 Union at Ice House Alley/Sansome & Battery.

2 Union at Sansome.

3 Vallejo/Montgomery & Kearny.

1 Vallejo at No. 474/Montgomery & Kearny.

1 Vallejo/Sansome & Battery at Cowell.

TWIN PEAKS

A focal point for the entire city, as outlined in the 1905 Burnham Beautification Report whose ideas were discarded in the mad rush to rebuild after the 1906 earthquake and fire.

RATING

2 Burnett at Hopkins to Upper Burnett to Gardenside at No. 120.

4 Clayton at Corbett. View.

3 Clayton & Market.

3 Copper/Graystone & Corbett, next to No. 301 Graystone & No. 592 Corbett.

4 Corbett at No. 670 to No. 660.

4 Crestline at Twin Peaks Blvd.

2 Cuesta Court.

3 Cuesta Court, No. 42 to Corbett.

2   Fredela Lane/Clairview Court & Farview Court.

2   Fredela Lane/Lower Marview & Clairview Court.

2   Glendale at Corbett.

3   Iron Alley/No. 495 Corbett & No. 1499 Clayton, with an extension
    to Graystone.

1   Market, opposite No. 3801.

1   Market/Romain & Glendale.

5   Pemberton Place/Crown & Clayton.

5   Twin Peaks.

3   Twin Peaks Blvd., next to No. 192, opposite Crown Terrace up to Tank Hill.

4   Twin Peaks Blvd. (lower) to Twin Peaks Blvd. (upper), opposite the end
    of Midcrest.

3   Twin Peaks at Christmas Tree Pt. vista.

2   Vista Lane/Burnett at No. 535 to Gardenside to Parkridge to
    Crestline at No. 70.

UPPER MARKET

This neighborhood is enjoying a renaissance. Community groups are
renovating gardens and houses.

RATING

2   Ashbury/No. 57 & No. 81 Ashbury Terrace. Seven small stairways be-
    tween street and sidewalk.

4   Ashbury Terrace, next to No. 64. 1911–1912 development.

2   Clifford Terrace at Roosevelt No. 475, to Lower Terrace No. 180. Round-
    ing a corner and continuing across the street.

4   Corbett, next to No. 334. Very steep alley, with stairway and walkway to
    1310 Clayton.

1   Corbett & 17th St. The two steps serve the purpose of rounding the
    corner.

3   Corbin Place/No. 200 Corbett & No. 4399 17th St.

3   Danvers/18th St. & Market. A 1946 stairway.

3   Douglass/States & 17th St. Charming, tree-lined cul-de-sac, with an
    assortment of Victorians.

3   Levant/States & Roosevelt. High retaining wall covered with vines.
    Butterflies and chickadees abound in the foliage. Curbed street com-
    plements stairway.

3   Lower Terrace & Saturn.

1   Ord Court at No. 2 to Douglass cul-de-sac. Surprise.

3   Ord/Storrie & Market, down to Ord at 18th St. Happy wall mural on
    No. 176 Ord at end of stairway.

2 Roosevelt at 17th St. Rounding a corner.

3 Saturn/Lower Terrace and top of Saturn Stwy. Seven useful stairways interacting with sidewalk and street.

2 Saturn at No. 154/Temple & Roosevelt. One three-step stairway.

4 Saturn/end of Saturn & Ord. Redesigned by Department of Public Works. Benches and planted areas augment curving stairway.

2 17th St. & Mars. Rounding a corner.

3 Upper Terrace. Monument Way at 17th Ave./Clayton & Roosevelt, to Upper Terrace. View. You're at the geographical center of San Francisco.

4 Upper Terrace. No. 480 at Mt. Olympus down to Upper Terrace No. 227. View. Neighborly.

3 Upper Terrace. Steps to Mt. Olympus monument.

5 Vulcan/Levant & Ord. Caring neighbors and cobblestone— not to be missed.

VISITACION VALLEY

Lively mix of ethnic cultures and neighborhood participation.

RATING

3 Beeman Lane/Wabash & San Bruno.

3 Campbell/San Bruno & Bayshore.

5 Campbell/Elliot & Visitacion Ave. Unexpected, long, in open-space setting.

3 San Bruno to Bayshore Blvd., near Arletta. See the inscription "Safety Subway" on the concrete wall of corner staircase.

5 Visitacion Valley Greenway/Leland & Tioga. Unusual setting.

2 Ward/Girard at No. 95 & San Bruno.

WESTERN ADDITION

This neighborhood survived the 1906 earthquake and grew and grew until it reached its peak during World War II.

RATING

3 Alamo Square. Fulton at Pierce, into square.

3 Alamo Square. Fulton at Steiner, into square.

3 Alamo Square. Grove at Scott, into square.

3 Alamo Square. Grove at Steiner, into square.

3 Alamo Square. Hayes at Pierce, into square.

2 Alamo Square. Hayes/Scott & Pierce. Divided street, four separate stairways.

4 Cottage Row at Sutter to Bush/Webster & Fillmore.

3 Koshland Park. Page at Buchanan, into park. Seven small stairways on path through park.

2   Pierce/Duboce Park & Waller.

2   Steiner/Geary & Post. Stairway to skyway over Geary.

YERBA BUENA ISLAND

Part of imperial San Francisco. Entry is the first exit on the Bay Bridge traveling east.

RATING

2   Lower Yerba Buena Road to Upper Yerba Buena Road. Stairway and path.

3   Macalla Court to Yerba Buena Road. Stairways and path.

1   Macalla Road under Bay Bridge. Relic stairway with steel railing in the middle of nowhere.

2   Macalla Road at Yerba Buena Road. Connects to path along road.

2   Yerba Buena Road at Forest Road. Old concrete stairway to nowhere; used to connect to path to summit.

CONSERVATIVE COUNT OF STAIRWAYS

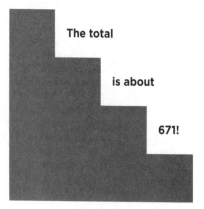

The total

is about

671!

Index

About the Authors

ADAH BAKALINSKY grew up in St. Paul, Minnesota, surrounded by flat land. She remembers trying, as a child, to walk up icy Ramsey Hill (near Pleasant Avenue) in winter, slithering down, trying again, and finally reaching the top. Fifty years later, while walking the old neighborhood on a visit, she discovered a stairway had been built to ascend the hill!

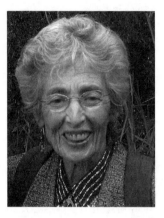

photo by Kate Brock

Looking for a synthesis for her social work, music, and film background, she discovered, surprisingly, that it was walking. She walks and, as she walks, she talks to whomever will talk with her. She carries a tape recorder to capture stories; she finds that walks shape themselves into a variety of musical forms and dances, and she redesigns a walk until it has just the rhythm it must have. She walks to see and returns to photograph the objects that give flavor to the walk. She feels lucky to live in San Francisco, where walking seems the most natural way to traverse the City.

Happy heeling, frisky footing, and merry walking!

MARY BURK has been walking the stairways of San Francisco since the 1980s. While researching the city and its seven hills, Mary discovered Adah Bakalinsky's book and quickly fell in love with her unique way of bringing the city to life.

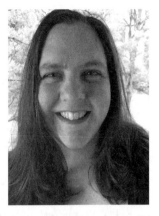

Mary and Adah first met at a book event for the fourth edition at the San Francisco Main Public Library. The two became fast friends, bonding through their deep interest in exploring the city on foot. Adah shared with Mary how every walk has its own rhythm, and so the two of them began improvising new walks together. Three editions later, Adah has passed the torch to Mary. But Mary and Adah still walk together and scout out new stairways and interesting routes for upcoming editions. When not out walking, Mary works as a software systems consultant and enjoys swimming and cooking. She shares a home with her husband, their two cats, and their 15-year-old catfish.

photo by Jason Heffel

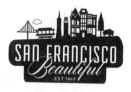

San Francisco Beautiful

San Francisco Beautiful was founded in 1947 by Friedel Klussmann in the course of her successful campaign to save the City's fabled cable cars. The organization's stated mission is to create, enhance, and protect the unique beauty and livability of San Francisco. It encourages and rewards citizen activism through its coveted annual Beautification Awards, works with civic leaders and community organizations to promote healthy and sustainable urban planning and design policies, and facilitates neighborhood-improvement projects. Preserving and restoring the City's public stairways and stairway gardens is of particular interest to the organization.

People interested in supporting San Francisco stairways and other neighborhood-improvement projects, and San Francisco residents looking for assistance in improving their neighborhood stairways, should visit **sfbeautiful.org.**

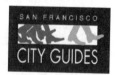

San Francisco City Guides

San Francisco City Guides is a volunteer organization that gives more than 60 free walking tours throughout the City, including walks on San Francisco stairways. Since 1978, City Guides have been leading these informative tours of San Francisco's history, architecture, legends, and lore. These tours are sponsored by the San Francisco Public Library. For more information on participating in a City Guides walk or becoming a volunteer, visit **sfcityguides.org.**

Check out this great title from
Wilderness Press!

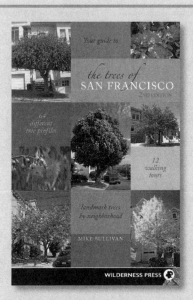

The Trees of San Francisco

By Mike Sullivan   6 x 9, paperback
ISBN: 978-0-89997-743-0   192 pages
$19.95, 2nd Ed   Color photos throughout

The Trees of San Francisco introduces readers to the rich variety of
trees that thrive in San Francisco's unique conditions. San Francisco's
cool Mediterranean climate has made it home to interesting and unusual trees from all over the world–trees as colorful and exotic as
the city itself. Light on botanical and scientific detail and jargon,
this book is designed to appeal to the general public and introduce
the average reader to the urban forest in one of America's most interesting cities. The book contains 12 neighborhood walking tours
infused with an "only in San Francisco" charm.

WILDERNESS PRESS
... on the trail since 1967

Check out this great title from
Wilderness Press!

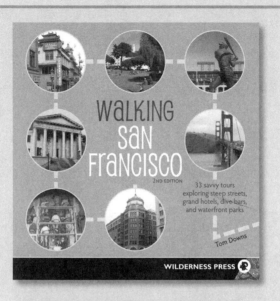

Walking San Francisco

By Tom Downs
ISBN: 978-0-89997-654-9
$18.95, 2nd Edition

7 x 7, paperback
248 pages
2-color

Walking San Francisco explores the best of the City "on the ground" with walks that traverse its length and breadth, from North Beach to Lands End, Glen Park to Golden Gate Park.

The 33 specially designed urban treks are not only good exercise but are a great way to soak up the history, culture, and vibe of the City by the Bay. The walks commentary includes trivia about architecture, local culture, and neighborhood history, plus tips on where to dine, have a drink, or shop. Each tour includes a clear neighborhood map and vital public transportation and parking information. Route summaries make each walk easy to follow, and a "Points of Interest" section lists each walk's highlights.

WILDERNESS PRESS
... on the trail since 1967